Dedicated to my mother, Jill Bruce

There you go mum.

Tangible evidence; it's not all in your head.

Introduction

This book is number 2 in The Secret Healer Series. It follows on from *The Complete Guide To Clinical Aromatherapy and Essential Oils of the Physical Body* (free on most e-book platforms) which details what an essential oil is and how it can help to mend a poorly body.

Consider that book to be the First Aid Kit, whereas *this book* is the start of the healing. Here we begin to understand the full majesty of how wondrous plant medicine is, but more importantly how incredible human physiology is. What is most amazing, is our bodies are perfectly made to heal themselves through the scents of essential oils affecting changes in the brain, but this can be even more improved by massage.

The ethos of complementary medicine has always been that we are not singularly a physical body, but that we also are affected by our emotions and our spiritual wellness too. Until very recently this was considered the right-on vision of the hippy fraternity, but remarkable new discoveries into the biochemistry of neuroscience has suddenly jet propelled aromatherapy into a whole new dimension of healing.

Scientists believe the brain's mood drug serotonin, may play a huge part in our fight against disease, greatly enhancing a person's capability to fight cancers, reduce diabetes and prevent heart attacks and strokes. What's more they now know that our magical essences, not only make you feel good, this energy vitally kickstarts the body's immunity to safeguard and heal it. If you think our delicate essential oils are airy fairy, think again. These aromatic oils are fierce warriors of healing ready to annihilate germs and pathogens or shadows lurking at the back of the mind.

For millions of people the cream and pills from the doctor will suffice. They will stop their itching and chase away the night monsters that haunt their dreams. Hallelujah for that, too.

But...there are still billions of others who have not yet achieved happiness, let alone wellness. If you are one of those people, or you come into contact with them in a work or personal relationship, then this book is for you.

Come with me, together let's slay emotional dragons, overpower monsters that haunt your dreams, chase away the terrors likely to be causing your illnesses....

And enter a world of calm.

Because, right here, right now....

This could be the first day of your *longer* life.

Table of Contents

Introduction 2

Table of Contents 4

The Triangle of The Mind Body and Spirit.................9

Our Sense of Smell and How It Affects Our Brain 11

The Limbic System...11

Olfactory Pathways 15

The Connection Between the Mind Body Spirit 25

The Ancient Wisdom of the Mind, Body, Spirit............31

The Aura..31

The Chakras 33

The Science of the Mind Body Spirit - The Bodymind...........45

The Building Blocks of Life 46

Receptors..46

Ligands..47

Neurotransmitters 47

Steroids 48

Peptides 48

The Chemical System Nervous System 49

Neuropeptides – The Molecules of Emotion 52

Agonist and Antogonist 53

The Mobile Mind 54

    Its role in disease 54

    Vibration 58

The Mind Body Connection....................................61

    Pain Relief..64

Emotions and The Organs 66

    Liver 67

    Gall bladder 69

    Kidneys 70

    Heart 72

    Spleen 74

    Stomach 75

    Bowels..76

    Lungs..77

    Skin 79

    Genitals 80

    Blood 80

    Immunity 81

    Peak Flow of Organs...82

Part 2 - The Holistic Principle 84

Mind Body Spirit Principle 85

The Spirit 85

Give Me Joy In My Heart...89

Part 3 The Healing 97

Meditation 97

Hypnosis 99

Essential oils for chakra healing................................99

Crown...100

Brow...100

Throat 100

Heart...100

Solar Plexus 100

Sacral 100

Base or root 101

The Emotions...101

Anger 106

Irritation 107

Exasperation 107

Rage 108

Disgust 108

Envy 109

Torment 109

Sadness 109

Suffering 110

Sadness 110

Disappointment 111

Shame 111

Sympathy 112

Fear 112

Horror 112

Nervousness 113

Trust 114

Love 114

Affection 115

Lust 115

Longing 116

Joy 116

Cheerfulness 116

Zest 117

Contentment..117

Pride 118

Optimism..119

Enthrallment 119

Relief...119

    Surprise 120

    Contraindications of this section....................120

Conclusion..121

About the Author...123

Other Works by The Author 125

Disclaimer..138

The Triangle of The Mind Body and Spirit

Hugs, not drugs....

Isn't that what they say? It is a powerful statement; but what, actually, does it mean?

Perhaps it means that feeling loved is the key to being well?

Maybe it refers to the healing power of touch.

Could it mean that, often, there is a better way to wellness than reaching for the medicine cabinet?

Five thousand years ago, the ancient texts, The Vedas, were given to the sages. Contained within, were truths about an extraordinary system of energy existing inside and outside of our bodies. This chakra system now forms the basis of Ayurvedic medicine, yoga and Tibetan Buddhism as well as many other branches of religion and healing. These wheels of energy, complete with the aura were believed to be mechanisms of emotional and physical wellness. Until recently though, this New Age philosophy had no scientific basis to back it up.

In the late 20th Century a piece of research, nominated for the Nobel Prize for Science was to become the foundation for proof of the bumper sticker philosophy that had been touted for thousands of years. In the 35 years that have followed, the entirely new science of psychoneuroimmunology has formed and blossomed. At last we have proof that complementary medicine has always been correct in its assumptions that our state of mind affects our health. What's more, not only can we affect our health through our thoughts by interceding and altering them, but the very simplest form of this alchemy can be concocted using essential oils.

Psychoneuroimmunology

It's definitely not a word you would want to get in your spelling test, right? In fact, it is so new that the spell-checker in Word does not recognise it and when I upload this book to Amazon, the automatic proof reader will likely throw it up as an error too.

Nevertheless, ground breaking scientists in this field are squirreling away, feverishly trying to discover how our thoughts can affect our health. It relies on a three-way collaboration in the body, that **_psycho_**logy sets off **_neuro_**logical changes in the body, which in turn can affect our **_immun_**ity.

The physiology of this is explained in far more detail in chapter 3, but our quest is an exploration into how **_aromatherapy_** plays a part in this. In _The Complete Guide to Clinical Aromatherapy and Essential Oils of the Physical_

Body, I explained there were two routes for essential oils to heal the body. They are absorbed through the skin and into the blood stream and they also travel up the nose, via the olfactory nerves and affect a part of the brain called the limbic system. Let's begin by getting a better understanding of exactly what the limbic system *is* and what it *does*.

Our Sense of Smell and How It Affects Our Brain

The Limbic System

The limbic system is complex set of structures found in the brain, just under a section called the cerebellum. It was discovered, accidentally, by James Olds and Peter Milner in 1954.

Their initial discovery arose when they were stimulating rats with electrical impulses. The animals, very quickly learned ways to press the lever themselves, in order to trigger the same sensations. Soon, the rodents were sending electrical charges, to themselves, many thousands of times an hour.

It is believed by many that *emotional response* happens in the limbic system. It is thought to be the seat of each of our pain, anger, hunger, sex, thirst, and pleasure responses. Memories are also believed to be formed and stored here. We still know very little about how the brain works and so each time a new discovery is made about a function, there is reason for great celebration! Progression, in this field is so swift, that potentially, in 12 months time, the research in this book will be completely outdated. As the author, that truth is dreadfully frustrating, but as a healer I greet it with excited enthusiasm. Here are some of the things we *do* know about the system.

There are several areas of the brain that contribute to the process.

Long term memories are formed in the ***hippocampus***.

Pleasure and fear trigger the ***amygdala*** via a mechanism called the ***pleasure pathway*** through its **rewards system**.

The amygdala particularly comes into play in mating, but also in recall. It is also the mechanism that helps a person to remember minute details of their surroundings at any given time. You might consider how accurately a person can recollect details of a crime (fear triggers) or conversely the first time they met their lover (pleasure triggers).

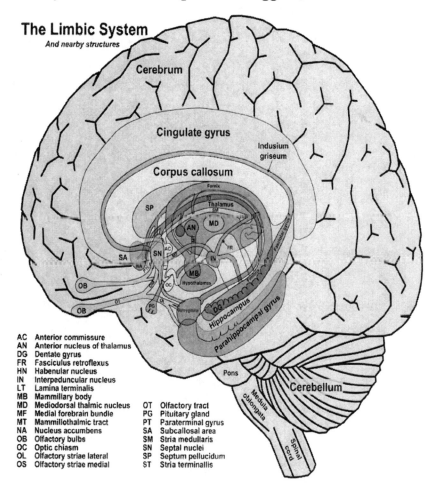

The Limbic System
And nearby structures

Cerebrum

Cingulate gyrus

Indusium griseum

Corpus callosum

Fornix

SP

Thalamus

AN   MD

AC

FR

SA   SN

MB

OC   Hypothalamus

OB

DG

OB

Hippocampus

Parahippocampal gyrus

Pons

Cerebellum

Medulla oblongata

Spinal cord

AC	Anterior commissure		
AN	Anterior nucleus of thalamus		
DG	Dentate gyrus		
FR	Fasciculus retroflexus		
HN	Habenular nucleus		
IN	Interpeduncular nucleus		
LT	Lamina terminalis		
MB	Mammillary body		
MD	Mediodorsal thalmic nucleus	OT	Olfactory tract
MF	Medial forebrain bundle	PG	Pituitary gland
MT	Mammilliothalmic tract	PT	Paraterminal gyrus
NA	Nucleus accumbens	SA	Subcallosal area
OB	Olfactory bulbs	SM	Stria medullaris
OC	Optic chiasm	SN	Septal nuclei
OL	Olfactory striae lateral	SP	Septum pellucidum
OS	Olfactory striae medial	ST	Stria terminallis

13

Recognition and recollection is controlled by the **mammillary body**, and some scientists believe this actually forms part of the **hippothalamus** too. When you recognise a person, or a place, then the mammillary body is being activated.

The **limbic node** seems to work separately from the rest of the system and can be further dissected into three more parts.

- **Parahippocampal gyrus**: This processes spatial memory. It is vital to learning and reasoning and is also what helps you to recognise your immediate environment.
- The **Cingulate Gyrus** has mental and physical functions. It controls our cognitive and attentional processing of thoughts. Physiologically, it also regulates our heart rate and blood pressure.
- The **Dentate Gyrus** is believed to be involved in the formation of any new memories we create.

Many scholars also consider the **Entorhinal Cortex** and **Piriform Cortex** to, also, be part of the limbic system. These play a valuable part in the pleasure pathway and are fundamentally involved in the processes causing a person to develop an addiction.

Decision making happens in the ***Orbito-frontal Cortex***. How effectively this part of the brain processes, will influence a person's level of aggression but also their learning abilities.

Is it just me, or is that really fascinating?!

Clearly, then for essential oils to start affecting these sectors of the brain, we need to get them there in the first place. You will remember that certain parts of an essential oil are able to pass through the blood brain barrier. Some of the essential oils, absorbed through the skin, will find their way to the limbic system. But, there is a faster route though, isn't there?

Yup, up your nose! So how does that work? Well the first thing to know is...the effects happen very quickly. There is only one electrical connection (synapse) between the nose and the brain.

Olfactory Pathways

In fact, the molecules of the oil go along two routes, if you think about it. When you breathe in air containing odorant molecules, they can also enter the body through your mouth. They travel to the brain, this time via the pharynx. The nasal route is referred to as the ***primary pathway,*** and if they travel through the mouth, we say they have gone along the ***secondary pathway***.

In the nasal cavity, molecules are projected onto the *Nasal Conchae*, then they reach the *Olfactory Mucosa*. This is where the magic happens. This tiny space in the nasal cavity, only measures about the size of a 5p piece (a dime, for my transatlantic friends) and is like a carpet of receptors cells. In this minute cavity, are no fewer than 100 million receptors. This remarkable part of our anatomy is the reason we enjoy such an inordinately comprehensive sense of smell.

Proteins and receivers are contained within tiny finger-like protrusions called cilia. Their job is to catch the air as it passes them, and then read the messages they receive. They, then, send minute electrical signals along the cilia to two structures called the **glomeruli** and the **olfactory bulbs**.

These olfactory bulbs are actually in two parts, the left and right bulbs, and form small outcroppings of the brain. They are just behind the basal lobe and are made up of many different layers, each one contacted by hundreds of fibres. Every fibre has its own job of carrying messages along this pathway.

To this stage, the process is quite well understood, but the next parts are still subject to many investigations. It is thought that messages run from the *lateral olfactory tract* to the *primary olfactory cortex*. Messages are then transported through the **thalamus** and then receptors are triggered in the **orbito-frontal cortex**. This is where, it is thought, that our perception of smell is triggered. Smell then, seems to happen somewhere between the thalamus and the amygdala.

In *The Professional Stress Solution* we look very closely at how the amygdala processes memories and, in turn, stress. The job of the amygdala is to translate memories and thoughts into images. This means you are able to conjure pictures of lavender when you smell it.

Now, if this was any other aromatherapy book, I would say this is why lavender oil might remind you of your grandmother, jasmine of a beautiful holiday, or even the smell of baking bread might make you smile. All of these are true, and potentially form some of the reasons aromatherapy is so popular. But those of you who have read more of my work know that The Secret Healer is not really that interested in the hearts and flowers of essential oils. There are plenty of other books to teach you that. I love them because they are healers and so to investigate this I want to look at the connection of smell and memories from a darker slant; from that of PTSD.

For some people, this processing can become a living hell. For people suffering from Post-Traumatic Stress Disorder, memories get stuck, in transit, before being placed into storage, in the mind. These pictures remain in a perpetual repeat loop, transporting a person back to the same place over and over again.

In a moment, you will read a powerful passage where a soldier relates how smells affect his everyday life. Here, Joseph Miller speaks of how memories of Iraq are triggered by everyday scents. I will warn you: this is a harrowing piece and so feel free to jump over it if you feel you cannot take it. It is a mesmerizingly graphic account of the smells of war and human loss, and how, in some ways, he is not ready to let go of that. I cry all the way through it, every time I read it. I want, however, to demonstrate just how powerful a link there is between smell and wellness.

Jo relates

"As a platoon leader I was ready to lead my soldiers, even in the most trying of circumstances, but when I arrived to the aftermath of a suicide bomber detonated on a crowd of civilians I wasn't prepared for the smell. In my experience blood doesn't have a smell at first, although it is very visible, tends to flood your memory and when it stains clothing that smell imprints itself on the memory event as it were there in the moment. In honesty that street corner mostly smelled like

dirt and dust, because the explosion had picked it up off of the ground. The smell of explosives was present, I was used to those smells, but the smell of burning flesh was much more apparent and different then anything I had ever experienced (still this was muted by the overwhelming smell of scattered dirt and dust). The smell of burned flesh was like smell of burnt hair, yet exponentially grown by the scale of that terrible day in northern Iraq. This mixed with the smell of burning meat, though completely unappetizing and unseasoned. The only way I can describe the smell of peoples skin is that it was as if leather was left out in the rain long enough to fester slightly, and then it was burned, or at least how I image that would smell. The addition of the burnt clothing created an earthy smell, which was a mixture of burning leaves and grass/marijuana.

Still, no matter how traumatic the stench of death and violence was I mostly inhaled the terrible smell common in the urban centers of Iraq created by the burnt trash, raw sewage flowing through the streets, and the awful smell that the dirt and dust made as it lodged itself into your nasal passages. A not so insignificant part of the awful smell of Iraq was my body odor, because I lived in an outpost and showered weekly at best. Only that day the smell of Iraq was amplified by an explosion that wafted it through the air.

Despite the stench, I refused to throw away my flesh stained boots, because I would spend a lifetime, if necessary, walking that smell away. After nine years and thousands of miles it is still there in my boots, so are the bloodstains, and the barbwire scratches I got rushing to that intersection on another night. That smell has also stained my very being as an unmovable and unalterable weight on my memory. Even during exercise my sweat pours more profusely than it did before and rather than overpowering the stench of that day the sweat contributes to it as if my every pore was endeavoring to recreate the smells of that moment. Stress sweat is more pungent than normal thermal regulatory perspiration. My body remains attached to the muted ammonia smell of muscle deterioration that comes with the body's processing of the stress chemical cortisol. I have smelled fresh cow brands and had a terrible panic attack. Anytime I smell burning hair, unseasoned meat, grass, warm sewage in a portable toilet, marijuana or the dust of the desert I am back there again: only naked, unarmored, helpless, and alone. My heart races and I can't seem to breath.

The stench combined with the chaotic sights, sounds, my internal dialogue, and physical sensations, though the smell was by far the worst of all my sensations that day (well that and feeling the weight and limpness of a dead flesh). Smells today are forever different and can send me into PTSD symptoms, often simply sicken me, or worst give me terrible migraine headaches. A lifetime of therapy and doing the right things to manage PTSD will never make that memory less burdensome. Although, I am still proud that I have refused to get rid of those boots because they are like my tattoos, a symbol of my commitment to deal with the violence I witnessed: to face my PTSD. Preserving my boots, even if they still smelled like that day in the hopes of walking them clean, was the first gesture of my efforts to face my burdensome memories no matter how terrible, with as much honor and strength as possible. The smells are certainly less pungent now, and the memory is too, at least with every attempt to understand and accept them. As if taking the time to remember that awful stench, or any sensation for that matter as it was, or as they were, reduces their terrible grasp on my life..."

Are you still with me? Feel like you have been ripped to shreds? What a brave man.

So, we know a smell can trigger memories. It will cause the limbic system to kick into response and act in unusual ways. It not only triggers emotions but also primal instincts, whether that is to run from danger, but also to eat or procreate too.

But clearly smell can also affect the emotions too (via the limbic system), and emotions most certainly affect our quality of life. How many times have you gone off your food because something upset you (or actually because you were madly in love too). If you are in a bad mood, tender lovemaking is most probably off the menu.

When you visit an aromatherapist then, he or she will probably ask you to smell the oils to check you like them, but more because of the associations it will bring forward for you in your therapy. The interesting thing is, most certainly you will perceive the smell of an oil in a very different way to anyone else.

I have a vivid memory of being about 12 and walking home from school becoming very irate with my friends because I could not make my thoughts clear to them about the colour green. It was autumn, and the grass was a deep lush emerald hue, but I had become engrossed with the question "How can I know they see the same green as me?" I had no point of reference to know if perhaps their green was what I knew as red, and for weeks it really bothered me. Then Duran Duran released a new single and that strange vexation was gone! Years later though, my son introduced me to an idea called Qualia, and the strange thought was back. This time, though, I was relieved to find I was not alone in wondering it.

In 1947, it seems the eminent neuro expert Daniel C. Dennett, also had the same ponderings as me and described qualia as "an unfamiliar term for something that could not be more familiar to each of us: *the way things seem to us*."

There is still debate as to whether qualia does exist, but it remains a truth that whilst the anatomy of your nasal cavity is likely to be identical to mine, I may hate some essential oils that you love. Do they, in fact, smell the same to me, or am I *experiencing* them in a different way?

In some cases, there is a specific genetic reason for this, though. I love coriander, it is fresh, zingy and spicy, but my husband hates it. He says it tastes and smells like soap. He is right...and he is wrong. Scientists have identified the gene OR6A2 translates our perception of aldehydes in tastes and smells, and it is this factor that makes people divisive over fresh and zingy versus soapy. This difference of genetic coding is just one reason for the difference of experience. Memory as we have seen is another.

The difference that makes the difference....

Because, ain't that the truth? No two of us is completely identical. In a million, jillion, squillion, bjillion and six ways, (I asked my five year old what's the biggest number he could come up with! Not sure why he never made it to seven...) we are different. Genetically, socially, psychologically and culturally...I am different to you. Your emotional triggers will be separate to mine.

And yet, incredibly, it seems certain emotions bring up the same illnesses over and over again. How can that be? Anybody would think it was chemical.....

Hmmm, hold that thought.

The Connection Between the Mind Body Spirit

When you visit the doctor, he will listen to your description of your symptoms and provide a treatment designed to treat just *that one* thing. So, you might tell him you have eczema and he will give you a salve to treat the redness and itching. He might also give you another treatment that will heal where the skin has become broken too. The sufferer of IBS might be given something to try to calm their bowels, or the insomnia sufferer, a treatment to help them sleep.

In each case, a good doctor will ask if there seems to be any particular trigger that sets the flare off. In most cases they will also address diet and stress.

In the confines of the doctor's surgery though, appointment times make it impossible for the doctor to delve further into the symptoms themselves. And that is where a complementary practitioner excels. Our job is to look at the prevailing skin condition, stomach complaint or sleeplessness and ascertain whether it might be purely the top layer of something far more complex.

The doctor is absolutely correct in his assumption that stress is likely to be underlying factor. But, clearly, my stress is very different to yours. You might look at me in utter confusion if I get upset about something, and wonder "what on earth's got in to her". Our psychology as humans is utterly complex, wrapped up in our familial history, societal constraints and of course, our temper on any particular day.

Again, it's the difference that makes the difference.

The extraordinary thing is our bodies read these emotions and turn them into physical symptoms. On closer examination, we find it is often the same set of feelings being exhibited every time that same illness rears its head. To the patient, this can seem ridiculous, because looking at illness from the top down it might seem there is no common thread. But, once you start to understand which emotions press which physiological buttons, it makes you look at the illness in a different light. Naturally, this means you can also begin to take control.

The complementary practitioner then, takes a more holistic approach. That is, he looks at the symptom purely as one tiny piece of the jigsaw of a person's life. He looks at many different dimensions of the person's being, to see where that original trigger might be coming from. He will examine the patient's diet, her lifestyle, how she feels about her work, her family life, her relationship with her parents and siblings and their general demeanour too.

Examining the mind, body and spirit might seem like there are three different areas of a person, and in some ways that is so.

More often though, you can see the three sides are entirely interdependent on each other; almost like that 3D optical illusion triangle. (Penrose Triangle) Where did it start and where does it finish.

Consider this:

Patient A has a very well paid highflying job.

She has loved her job for many years and is extremely good at it. Three years ago she took a break to have a child and has returned after maternity, relieved to find she can still perform her duties as well as she ever did.

After about six months, though, she is finding her child needs more and more attention. She wants to play with him before she puts him to bed. That hour given to the child, means one less hour in front of spreadsheets and charts. She is tired, but determined and so she continues to put in the hours.

As the stress starts to rise she finds it harder and harder to switch off, and finds a glass of wine really helps. One, runs to two on really bad days, and this affects the quality of her sleep.

She is tired, looks dreadful, her work is suffering and to make things worse some mornings she is hung-over too.

So my question to you then is: when she gets to work on Thursday, with yet another headache...what was the cause?

Is it emotional?

Well yes, I suppose. She is getting stressed because she can't perform at the same level she once could. She feels guilty for leaving her child. Potentially she feels angry at the injustice of the situation too.

Is it physical?

Certainly it is chemical because the wine is taking its toll. It is the liver's job to cleanse the system of alcohol and so that will be exhausted too. She is, frankly knackered and so that, most certainly, is a physical factor.

Is it spiritual?

Potentially, depending on her beliefs about what a mother should be able to do, it could be, yes. Was her mum available to do everything for her as a child? Perhaps she feels she should be able to, too. Does she still feel the need to be number one at work and always turn in perfect spreadsheets? How much time is there left for her to indulge *herself* at the end of the day? Is she doing *anything* at all in a day that fulfils her *own* basic needs?

It is a complicated list, and as you can see the emotional and spiritual often overlaps and later I shall explain the mechanisms that ensure the emotional and physical also do.

There is always this triad of mind, body and spirit in perpetual influence of each other.

I had always known this, right from studying my Advanced Diploma of Aromatherapy, where we focused a lot on the effects of anger but, really, then my understanding went into a cul-de- sac and got stuck there for several years.

Then my dad became very ill. At the same time, I turned 40, so the doctor called me in to his surgery to have my middle aged person's MOT. All the tests came back fine, even my predilection for cake had bypassed diabetes and cholesterol, unscathed. There was one test, however, that caused concern and that was my kidneys.

I was very frightened by the thought they might be failing, but all worries about dialysis were entirely negated by the terror of the oncoming death of my belovéd father. This dreadful cancer was eating him alive and the spirit of my lovely dad was nowhere to be found in that shell of pain housing his soul. I hated seeing the torture he was enduring and longed for his soul to be freed.

I was so relieved for him when he died. For me his illness had been far worse than his death. When I went for my kidney tests results later that month, they were completely normal.

Years later, I have learned the emotion that affects the kidneys is fear. We will cover this more, later in the book, but first I would like to talk about the mechanisms that transport these emotions or spiritual disturbances to the organs, thus setting up illness and physical disease. First we will look at the ancient wisdoms and then I will fasten it down with the latest developments and evidence from science.

The Ancient Wisdom of the Mind, Body, Spirit

The Aura

Ancient wisdom tells us that, rather than just being a physical body, we actually have seven bodies. As well as the one we all recognise we also have, what are called, **etheric bodies**. These are collectively referred to as **the aura**, which is a field of energy emanating out from the body.

You might see this drawn as rainbows around the body, because the layers of the etheric bodies change colour, each one having a very specific meaning in terms of the personality and life status of the body, but also their health at that time.

There are many people who can see these rainbows around everyone. As a child, I could; but I made a conscious decision to stop seeing them or "turn it off" when I was about 9 years old because I hated being different to other people. If you think of the beautiful icons of early Christianity, you will often see the Christ Child depicted with a halo around his head. This is a good representation of seeing a gold aura; that is a very saintly colour.

The aura is the seat of our spirit. It is like a barometer of our emotions, and it filters through information from our consciousness to our physical body. As we explore the spirit, and the book unfolds, you will come to recognise how a person already unconsciously knows when they are veering away from things that will make them happy, long before this is demonstrated through their physical health (and make no mistake this most certainly will happen).

The aura is an entire subject, in its own right, but I have chosen not to cover it here. I shall, instead, refer you to a book written by my mother who can see auras very clearly indeed! *The Aura by Jill Bruce* explains about each etheric body, what emotions and spiritual challenges are likely to show themselves in each body, and how disease moves through the layers. By the end of the book the reader not only understands the etheric bodies well but is able to draw a diagram of anyone's aura including their own.

The Chakras

There is a diagram to help you with this section. Download it at *buildyourownreality.com/chakra-chart*

The chakras are wheels of energy which emanate through the aura and connect it to the physical body. These vortices protrude through the body from the front to the back. They vitalise our organs and are affected by emotional distress.

There are 7 major chakras and 23 other minor ones. For the most part we work with the 7. They have specific locations and should vibrate on clear, bright colours. Chakras should open and close rhythmically and should be located down the central midline of the body, head to feet.

Disease will show if they are locked closed, impeding energy to the organs, or conversely if they jam open and allow energy to pour away. They can also get pushed off line. This can happen for many reasons but the resounding catalyst is largely emotion.

Their correct colours and alignments should be:

Root

Located: At the base of the tail bone

Is aligned to: Independence, money, food, survival, grounding

Vibrates on the colour: Red

The root chakra is what binds us to this earth, this particular worldly manifestation. It is about our opinions and beliefs about what we need to survive. It is thought that the first seven years of our life affects this chakra the most, as our upbringing affects our worldly beliefs.

In particular, this might relate to limiting beliefs about money, or even about advancement in general. In the most extreme example, we have all seen money turn some people into right nasty pieces of work...but what if, as a child you began to believe this was the *only* thing money could do. I can tell you now, that child will never grow into a person who is able to earn a decent living, because his own conscience tells him it bad.

Extend that to anything relating to survival, food in particular. But the root chakra is all about the boundaries we put up, too. It could be personal space boundaries which make it difficult to bond, or it could be moral and ethical boundary dilemmas too. The best example I can think of here, is a girlfriend realising her partner is dealing drugs. She stays with him because she can't afford to leave. If, regardless of her disgust at the chain of despair he causes, she remains, this would a root chakra issue, I think. Extreme, but it demonstrates the point.

34

Of all the issues though, you can expect this chakra to betray issues with parents and upbringing. Do they feel anger or as if they have unfinished business. Do they feel they may have been victims of emotional or physical neglect? What is their perception of how well their parents fulfilled their need to survive? Not only were they fed and clothed but do they feel like they bonded and were loved?

You can probably sum this up by saying the emotions and feelings they feel they have been denied, or are continuing to deny. Think of really violent criminal urges which can no longer be contained and, yes ,that would relate to unbalanced (or possibly *mal-formed* since we are talking about upbringing here) root chakra energy, but this is very extreme.

Physical disease you might find with problems with the energy of the root chakra are: Elimination problems such as constipation (note the can't-find-a-way-to get-out synchronicity?) Since it is to do with food, you might also think anorexia because of control – however when it comes to an addiction, that is sacral energy. Joint pain and lower back pain are particularly seen.

Sacral

Located: 2 ins below the navel

Is aligned to: Abundance, well being, pleasure and sexuality

Vibrates on the colour: Orange

So as we start to grow, then our spiritual awareness lifts up. This is the energy of the older child, not quite adolescent. It is about creativity, the birth of sexuality, control and again, money. Here though, think of all of these in the context of one's own individuality.

Blockages of this energy will be seen as what we might dismissively call playground tactics but of course, uncomfortable as it is to admit, very few of us actually grow out of them.

Think:

- Power plays
- Jealousy or envy
- Betrayal
- Control

Physical disturbances you might see associated with sacral chakra energy are:

sexual problems, in particular, impotence and frigidity, problems with the bladder and urinary tracts, and also issues in the large intestine.

Here, I think it is worth commenting on the chicken and egg situation between emotions and the chakras. Sometimes the depleted energy will lead to a specific emotion, in this case let's say playing power games. But, just as often, the emotion will mess with the chakra energy too. A person betrayed, may try to exert control and probably won't want to have sex. The chakra didn't cause the physical issue....it carried it. There is always this constant fluctuation and communication between the three, always interlocked and potentially all showing problems in one way or another...no one single catalyst.

Solar plexus

Location: About 2 ins above the navel

Is aligned to: Self confidence, self worth, responsibility

Vibrates on the colour: Yellow

You can view this chakra as the balance between a person's intellect and their intuition. It, very much, controls a person's capacity to act because it is the seat of self esteem and also of their personal power.

The reactions you might find here associated with stress are:

- Being afraid to move forward into a new situation (or a skill)
- Indecision about how to make a step forward – which life direction to take
- Low self esteem
- Over sensitivity to criticism
- Unable to accept blame and apportioning all blame on other people
- Very hot erratic tempers
- Incredibly judgmental attitudes
- Becoming aloof
- The need to always exert power
- Becoming too demanding

Of course, the same applies as with all the chakras, you can also look for emotions on the flipside. If chakra energy is depleted, you might also find they are not demanding enough, not getting angry enough, allowing others to exert too much power on them.

Further: the illnesses you might find associated with an imbalance in solar plexus chakra energy are:

Diabetes, hypoglycaemia, gall stones, nervousness, low energy, muscle cramps, stomach problems, narcissistic personality disorder and also liver complaints.

Heart

Located: Centre of the chest

Is aligned to: Love, joy, inner peace

Vibrates on the colour: Green

In health, the energy passes up through the chakras to the crown. As each stage of development evolves so the energy changes and, in fact, the wavelengths get higher too. For the heart chakra to function, the wisdom of the lower chakras must have been assimilated. For example, if you are denying your feelings, how can you feel joy? If you are feeling like a victim, how can you find peace?

Once the issues of the lower chakras have been aligned, then loving energy can fill the heart. Here we feel joy, importantly we can forgive. As we reach the development of the heart chakra we begin to look out of ourselves as to what the world can give. We are open to be loved and are balanced in our approach. This is the time when we learn to [re-]establish trust. Note the association between sadness and a heavy heart; the energy pulls the vibration down.

So elements you might look for with this chakra are:

- Bitterness
- Resentment

- Inability to forgive
- Sadness
- Grief

Physical disturbances you might expect to find with an imbalance of the heart chakra are: circulation problems, high blood pressure, shortness of breath, lung and chest complaints, and often you will find the depleted energy sucks vitality through the upper back resulting in pain between the shoulder blades too.

Throat

Located: As one would expect

Aligned to: Communication, expression, truth

Vibrates on the colour: Blue

By the time we get to the throat chakra we starting to find ways we can express what we want from life. We begin to explore how we can manifest the reality we desire. A balanced throat chakra makes our voice clear and bright, our words are resilient and come out just right. But if the energy is off, we can find words come out garbled or intelligible to hear. Our words can often stick and struggle to make it out to others ears.

Not just words though, it is any kind of expression. Working in the throat chakra can mean your water colour painting improves or even the way you dance. One thing I have noticed, when my throat chakra is off, is my rhythm and timing also goes awry.

The reason for this strange phenomenon might have something to do with the way the throat chakra melds the head and the heart. It is the seat of integrity. Do the words the mouth says reflect an accord between the heart and the head? Lying for example, does not. Swallowing your pride does not. Delivering news for the good of the company at the expense of the people does not. Perhaps then, the off-rhythm is that tiny little beat we miss as we check our truths.

So what ways might this manifest? Coughing, sore throats, starting to mumble, jitter, or even developing a stammer for some, are all classic indicators that something with the throat chakra might be amiss.

Problems with not expressing your truths through the throat chakra might lead to physical disturbances such as:

Sore throats and other disorders in the upper respiratory tract, ear problems (think: *no, I'm sorry, I just don't want to hear!*) problems with the oesophagus and also the cervical neck and spine. (*Think: I've had a gut full of this and it's all becoming a bit of a pain in the neck!)* In extreme cases these problems might also cause issues with the thyroid gland and the hypothalamus. In less acute cases you may find a fever also comes with throat problems, almost as if to purge.

How strange that the chakra connected with expression has the most obvious spoken clues!

Pineal

Located: At the brow between the eyebrows

Is aligned to: Imagination, intuition, ability to make decisions

Vibrates on the colour: Indigo

Now the pineal chakra is when things begin to become arcane. We know what this life has to offer and we have learned to accept it. Outside of this realm though, the pineal wants to know, what is there?

This is the seat of the third eye. It is seeing, in fact no, it is *knowing*.

When the energy of the third eye is activated, we discover intuition; we start to realise things we could not possibly know. We start to notice synchronicities and the events of our life start to flow.

Problems with this chakra can present as being delusional or lacking in insight. There is a lack of creative imagination and an inability to visualise.

Physical problems which might point to a disturbance in this chakra are:

Headaches, poor memory, neurological problems, in particular, with the pituitary and pineal glands.

Crown

Located: Above the head

Is aligned to: Our ability to connect with our spirituality, pure bliss

Vibrates on the colour: violet

This is the portal which connects us to consciousness. Energy flows down from creation through the crown chakra. So, then it becomes easier to see energy is a constant cycle of flux, from the root to the crown and out, in through the crown, down to the root and then back up again.

So then, this chakra can very easily be blocked either side, before inspiration enters, or after.

It is hard to say this chakra is aligned to emotion, more a state of mind of being open, being available for intuition to enter, having a high vibration of compassion, and of sending healing goodness out into the world.

I suppose, being healers, we move in the right circles to see this chakra blocked open more than many other people do. This is dissociative behaviour, spiritual obsession, having your head in the clouds. Be honest, you know you know someone!

By the same token, you might be looking for a lack of intuition or even having an unawareness of one's place in the universe.

Physical disorders you might be looking for are: migraine, mental health issues, amnesia and neurological disorders.

As a healer, seeing these correlations in a person's health never ceases to amaze me. Over and over, you see the same trends and patterns and it does make intervention to bring about healing much easier.

But the truth is, it is all a bit woowoo and out there, isn't it? Nebulous, intangible, a bit spooky and off the wall, or someone described it to me, not long ago...it is all very right on.

Well not any more. Now finally, we have the proof.

The Science of the Mind Body Spirit - The Bodymind

At the end of the twentieth century a neuroscientist named Candace Pert started to put together *medical* jigsaw pieces that could add meat to the bones of the idea that emotional and physical wellness were one and the same.

Pert had become an overnight star at just 26, when she had been able to locate and measure the opiate receptor in the body in 1972. Working in an extremely competitive lab at Johns Hopkins University, she had tried to explain how opiates such as morphine have such an extraordinary effect on the body. She wondered why the effects were not only limited to physically easing pain, but also markedly changing emotional states too, with their blissfully euphoric effects. She was able to identify the opiate receptor in the body as a molecule known as a peptide; her finding was to create the stepping stone for the discovery of the body's natural internal morphine that we today now know as endorphin. Later her work was to become instrumental in overturning how we view the neurological system today.

Looking back at my neurology notes from when I qualified in '93, it is extraordinary to see how much more we know about the nervous system in even that short amount of time. My notes, like most other peoples, show a sophisticated electrical circuitry of neurons, axons and dentrites running from the brain and through the body, mainly through the spinal column. We now know this is only half of an exquisite mechanism of, not only electrical impulses, but chemical ones too.

The Building Blocks of Life

When Pert had identified the opiate receptor she was able to demonstrate it was a beautifully elegant molecule which existed in parts of the body one would not ordinarily expect.

Receptors

A molecule is the smallest unit that can be found of a substance. Invisible forces attract and repel molecules allowing them to act in different ways. Receptors are in a constant flux of energy and are activated by something called a *ligand*. Initially ligands were described as being like keys fitting into locks (the receptor being the lock) however we now know that the molecules are actually continually wiggling and bouncing against each other, slipping on and off of each other and causing a vibration. When a ligand slides onto a receptor, it brings about changes in the body.

Ligands are made up of proteins. The very smallest building block of a protein is an amino acid. These amino acids are strung together, in tiny chains, almost like a necklace. The receptors act like sensory organs, consistently scanning the body and reacting on information they receive from the ligands.

Together the receptor and ligand work in harmony, which could be described as ringing the doorbell to open up the cell. The receptor, having received the message, sends it from the outer surface of the cell, into the cells interior. This can cause the state of the cell to change dramatically. From that signal, any number of changes happen in the body, all based on the action of that solitary ligand.

Ligands

There are three types of ligands. They are generally much smaller than the receptors they bind to. The binding of the receptors and ligands is extremely selective and specific. In other words only the right key will open the lock.

Neurotransmitters

You will recognise some of these neurotransmitters, I am sure. Histamine, the inflammatory chemical set off in allergic reactions (hence we use anti-histamines to reduce allergic reactions), dopamine, serotonin, norepinephrine, for example, are all neurotransmitters. Their function is to carry information across a gap in the communication of the cells called the synaptic cleft.

Neurotransmitters are the smallest of the ligands. They are found in the brain and in many other parts of the body.

Steroids

Again, many of these will be familiar to you, like oestrogen, progesterone, testosterone.

Peptides

The peptides form the largest number in the body. They consist of chains of 100 amino acids strung together, and under the microscope appear to be a little like a necklace turned in on itself. In total, they make up about 95% of the ligands found in the body. It helps to consider that if the cell is a machine then ligands are the buttons on the control panel, and the appropriate ligand is the finger that pushes the button and sets the cell into drive mode.

Since the initial discovery of the opiate receptor, many thousands of neuropeptides have been discovered and explored. We now know that:

Every peptide existing in bodily tissue is also found in the brain and vice versa.

Those neuropeptides originally thought to only exist in the brain were also found to be diffusing and binding throughout the body.

Every cell in the body is covered in millions of these receptors and is working almost like a satellite dish to pick up the right signal at the right time. The molecules are always in conversation, instructing the body what to do. Sometimes this might be "take up a bit more protein", or perhaps "stop dividing because we need more energy for digestion". Likewise it could be "Well that was embarrassing, open and close the blood vessels of the face, I think the big guy needs to blush" In the last example you can see a direct correlation between the thought, then the emotion and very swiftly after, physiological process.

Organs and glands have their own multi-directional communication network. They are consistently giving each other biofeedback as to how to achieve homeostasis. These molecules then, the peptides and neuropeptides are best termed as *information substances*, consistently chattering and vibrating through the body.

The Chemical System Nervous System

Nervous tissue is made up, mainly, from neurones which are highly specialised cells. The neurone has a *cell body,* which consists of a *nucleus* and *nerve fibres*. These fibres, branch out, extending as much as a meter away from the cell body. Long fibres called *axons*, carry signals *away* from the cell body. In turn, the shorter fibred *dendrite* carries them towards

49

the next cell body. A connection between two or more neurones is called a synapse.

The classical image of the nervous system then, was understood to be similar in function to a telephone system.

The brain sends a message to the bladder, for example. The instruction runs along the dendrite, along the axon and a synapse translates it to the nerve and then the body thinks "OOO, toilet quick" (Actually, it is getting my key out my pocket to open the front door that triggers this fastest, I think!) but it is now known that there is another part of this process that has been overlooked.

Neuropeptides and the synaptic gap

A colleague of Pert's at the National Institute of Mental Health (NIMH), Miles Herkenham, had been creating detailed maps of the electrical nervous system. His diagrams demonstrated there was a small gap between each of the synapses. This gap is what we have come to term as the synaptic cleft. So the question in his mind was "How is information being carried across these gaps?" He wondered if Pert's neurotransmitters might hold the answer.

Pert had already recognised, by this time, that the peptides were often found in clusters which she had referred to as hot spots or nodes. When she placed a diagram of the patches as she calls them, there were exact matches for the synaptic clefts, fitting identically into Herkenham's gaps. Working together Herkenham and Pert were able to map where neuropeptides were found in greatest number. They were able to ascertain locations of very high concentrations of the peptides, in intersections where a great amount of information

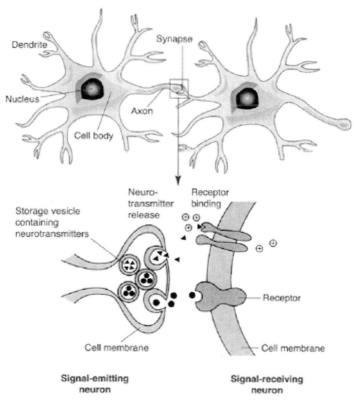

seemed to be required. She called these spots "Hot Spots or

"Nodes". It was supposed these worked as mini base camps sending information from local points in the body. *Fascinatingly, when she placed a diagram of the chakras over this map, she realised the seven biggest node conglomerations correlated exactly with the chakra locations.* Finally, alternative medicine had an explanation of how the emotions could vitalise the organs through the chakras.

Neuropeptides – The Molecules of Emotion

It is now recognised these patches are an essential part of our nervous system, not only filling the gaps between synapses in the body, but also in the brain. More important to notice, is their function then, not only happens in the brain, but throughout the body too.

Serotonin, for instance, is manufactured in the brain and the intestines. It is fundamental to mood balance and so we might expect its high concentration to be in the head however between 80-90% of the body's serotonin is found in the gastrointestinal tract. The rest is distributed between platelets and the central nervous system. This has massive ramifications for medicine, doesn't it? We now recognise the body doesn't simply exist to be a "stand" for the brain, holding the mind. It means the mind extends right through the body.

Agonist and Antogonist

Over the years, she replicated the same method to identify ligands as she had used that first time with the opiate receptor. It relied on the fact that each receptor required an *agonist* to activate it, or conversely an *antagonist* would prevent the ligand from entering the receptor and disallow any chemical reaction from taking place. In the initial experiment she had been using *naloxone*, the antidote doctors used against the effects of morphine. The initial question had been "why would a product, with an almost identical chemical structure to morphine, no longer cause a high or be relaxing. What was it that meant it had no effect? The answer, of course, was that the receptor did not recognise the substance and so the muscles and mind were not activated by it.

What is most fascinating about her tale (apart from the fact she was a woman excelling in the most misogynistic of fields, leading to the head of her lab being nominated for the Nobel Prize for the discovery of opiate receptor, instead of Pert herself being named) is how the establishment could no longer take her seriously, when she started to consider a seemingly "ridiculous" notion that these patches might be involved in *emotion*.

The Mobile Mind

On mapping the concentrations of these peptides it became clear our old perception of the emotional brain, that is the amygdala, hypothalamus and hippocampus operating as senior management from some detached penthouse suite, is not only out of date, it is radically incomplete. We can now see that rather than being a head housing a mind, above the neck, with the body separately below, we are in fact one mobile mind that extends right through the body.

Pert found that the place these nodes have the highest concentration is found within the limbic system. Interestingly these molecules can be found in massive quantities in the dorsal horn, one of the three columns of grey matter found in the spinal cord. This is the point of the first synapse of the nervous system where all of our bodily sensations are expressed. In fact, any location where there is an access to the senses finds a very high concentration of these molecules.

Its role in disease

It is believed that illness has the potential to take hold, spread and multiply because of a process called chemotaxis. Chemotaxis is the way a cell moves in response to a chemical stimulus. Somatic cells (that is: all cells in the body, apart from eggs and sperm) move themselves in response to chemicals within their environment, whether they move towards a receptor or away from it. In many conditions, there is much evidence to show serotonin (or 5-HT as it is more correctly known) influences whether allergenic or inflammatory receptors will be triggered in the body. What's more, serotonin (which is stored in the platelets of blood) actively triggers the release of neurophils in the system that fights infection.

Pert explains that although many illnesses, like cancers for instance, cannot be traced back to a negative emotion, the mindset has a great deal to do with how the body can come to fight it.

A cell has a natural cycle with checkpoints that help it to determine whether its current state is healthy and so therefore should divide, or whether it is damaged and so therefore should trigger cell death. Cancer can occur when the checkpoints go off kilter for some reason. In a healthy body, a powerful protein called P-53 triggers tumour suppression. Then, if damage is detected it causes a potential cancer to stop dead in its tracks.

A small percentage of cancers have genetic links, but many are thought to originate from toxicity from such factors as herbicides, petrochemicals and heavy metals and the patient's body is fervently trying to cleanse itself of this toxicity. Over time though, the large numbers of these, very healthy stem cells, begin to mutate and change into far more sinister cells.

Now, whilst this knowledge of toxicity means the cells don't relate to the emotion directly, Pert felt that the way they moved most definitely did, and chemotaxis held sway as to how this might happen.

In the video Miraculous Healings she gives an example where a woman has a difficult relationship with her brother, and she develops breast cancer. She suggests that the cells of the cancer would continue to secrete peptides that echoed her feelings connected with her brother. Over the years he had made her feel "I am worthless and insignificant" and these same emotions were rushing around her blood stream and being secreted by the cancer cells too. This would "convince" the cells of their need to grow and to feel bigger and more significant.

Simultaneously, she might have a realisation that, on the contrary, she was not worthless and the feelings of self-worth were directly related to her conflict with her brother and so therefore, external to her. This realisation, Pert suggests, has the power to stop the cancer growing. It activates the parts of the brain that control immunity, stimulates the bone marrow and spleen, releases killer cells, which in turn surrounds the cancer cell, and causes an inflammatory healing phase and then the tumour is gone. She ends by saying the Institute of Noetic Science has documentary evidence of thousands of cases where this has happened and cancer has been miraculously cured. Indeed trials are currently underway supporting the theory that the amount of serotonin in the blood affects how effectively P-53 triggers in our systems. These findings back up what alternative medicine had known for many years, that health and happiness are inextricably linked.

In 1985 Ed Blalock from the University of Texas found that a certain type of white blood cell, leukocytes, stimulated by a virus also secreted endorphins, as well as synthesizing its own identical version of ACTH. ACTH is a stress hormone made naturally in the pituitary gland, and its job is to stimulate the adrenal glands to release cortisol.

I cover cortisol at length in my book The Professional Stress Solution but in short its functions are:

- Blood sugar (glucose) levels

- Fat, protein and carbohydrate metabolism to maintain blood glucose

- Immune responses

- Anti-inflammatory actions

- Blood pressure

- Heart and blood vessel tone and contraction

- Central nervous system activation

What's important to note, now, is we have a very similar triangle of effects to that we saw in the Mind Body Spirit example at the beginning of the book.

A similar triangle now exists in the science that this is derived from, Psychoneuroimmunology (PNI). What did come first, the low emotion that caused the serotonin levels to drop, or the response to the viral invasion? You have the emotional aspect, the neurotransmitter transmitting the signals and then the immune response; and because this is a network of effects rather than simply being linear it means that any access for intervention come from a variety of points not least the place that changes the emotional triggers.

Vibration

It is amazing to me that Dr Pert explains that it is these vibrations of chemical reactions in the body that she thinks we experience as emotion, or indeed the energy we feel when we do healing of any description. William James wrote in 1884 that he believed emotions were visceral and so in turn, part of the body, rather than trickling down from the brain. Pert began to feel that this might be so. It is the collision of the molecules throughout our tissues that gives us butterflies in the tummy, for example. I don't know about you, but in times of real fear or heartache it has most definitely felt like a physical pain in my chest and stomach rather than something that emanated from my head?

She cites the research of Robert Plutchik, a psychology professor at Hofstra University.

His theory is we have **eight primary emotions**—these are:

- Sadness

- Disgust

- Anger

- Anticipation

- Joy

- Acceptance

- Fear

- Surprise

Experts agree emotions are transient. Moods are longer but still temporary, lasting hours or days. Personality though, is pretty much fixed.

These emotions, much like primary colors, could be mixed to create secondary emotions. For example:

- Fear + surprise = alarm

- Joy + fear = guilt

Naturally these do not switch from one to another, but rather become shades of one and less of another.

Emotions are what we experience when different peptides, neurotransmitters and hormones are released. She even goes on to explain she has been able to isolate one specific emotional and neuropeptide match.

Cortisone Releasing Factor (CRF) is made naturally in the hypothalamus. It is found in the spinal columns of suicide victims in ten times the concentration of other deaths. CRF1 is thought to be the receptor that triggers the feelings of euphoria when we drink alcohol. Studies are underway to try to create an antagonist of CRF1 to treat anxiety and also alcohol addiction. Pert describes CRF as being the neuropeptide of **negative expectations**. Later a work by Kent Berridge was to isolate **dopamine** as the **neurotransmitter of both desire and dread** (fascinating to think of the implication in the tremor of Parkinson's and the twitchiness of restless leg syndrome that is also now treated with dopamine). Depending on which part of the *nucleus* *accumbens* is stimulated, dictates which is felt; dread or desire. Amazingly, only a matter of millimetres makes the difference. In an experiment testing the affects of dopamine on rats secreting normal levels of the hormone, stimulating front of the nucleus accumbens caused the rats to eat three times as much as they would normally do. Stimulating the back caused them to act in a way they would when they encounter a predator.

The Mind Body Connection

Psychoneuroimmunology now has a recognised place in science and these findings have massive ramifications for health, especially through disciplines such as hypnosis and meditation but of course, for things like Law of Attraction too. We create what we are expecting. We can't really see things we have never seen before, so then visualisation now takes on an extremely important stance.

The brain is the head ganglion of the body. It tells the rest of the body what to do. If you believe in something really strongly enough, you *can* make it become a reality, she says. An extreme example is how our emotions literally guide our eyeballs and allow us to see what we are happy to see and filter out the rest. The *superior colliculous* in the dorsal part of the brain responds to motor and sensory signals, so this is the part of the brain that will instruct the eye to move to see a loud bang. In the same way, it can also stop the brain from processing the signals a husband cannot see when his wife is cheating, when everyone around him can clearly read the signs. The emotions prevent him from facing the truth.

She also proposes that the idea of the subconscious being in the head is also outdated and is better believed to be in the tissues of the body. As such when we experience great emotional traumas these are also integrated into the tissues. This can affect how well this part of the body performs or does not perform. In my opinion Caroline Myss portrays this best with her description of how "Emotional depth charges" affect our lives in the most remarkable ways.

Consider the effects of a soldier who has seen one of his men blown up beside him. How does this translate into the PTSD he sadly experiences when he returns home. Tests show these people excrete higher levels than usual of dopamine in their urine. The "fear" he experienced was dopamine coursing through his veins. The cell receptors were opened and cells throughout his body were flooded with dopamine. The "fear" remains right through his body.

If Pert is to be believed, it is not the counselling and psychiatry routes that bring about the greatest healing, but in fact, those that involve touch that release suppressed and forgotten emotions. Stretching, yoga, chiropractic and massage, she felt, were our greatest tools for healing.

Massage therapy and serotonin, dopamine and cortisol

In a 2005 paper produced by the Miami University School of Medicine, the effects of massage on hormones was monitored and reported.

The research reviewed studies on depression (including sex abuse and eating disorder studies), pain syndrome studies, research on auto-immune conditions (including asthma and chronic fatigue), immune studies (including HIV and breast cancer). It also reviewed studies on the reduction of stress on the job, the stress of aging, and pregnancy stress. In each case cortisol was tested either in saliva or in urine. The decrease of cortisol levels were significant (averaging decreases 31%).

Other studies monitored serotonin and dopamine in urine after massage. Here, an average increase of 28% was recorded serotonin and an average increase of 31% was noted for dopamine (remember dopamine is not only fear, but also desire).

Pain Relief

Now, if you think about it, the fact that any receptor in the body would respond to morphine, shows it was recognised by the body because a similar chemical existed naturally, whose objective was to trigger it organically. Soon after Dr Pert had found the opiate receptor, a Scottish team discovered the ligand that activated it. They termed it enkepaline. Later an American team were to claim their own part in the quest using the name endorphin, which is the name we recognise best today.

Endorphins floating around the system....what image does that give you? A buzz, a natural high, yes? In fact, later studies from Pert's lab would demonstrate to the world how strenuous exercise would trigger the phenomenon of "The runner's high", that allows him to carry on right through any pain barrier.

Proponents of the Natural Childbirth Trust and Lamaze will no doubt be cheering to know that endorphins are found in, and can be released from, the brain stem. And that breathing exercises and meditation bring about an altered state that allows us to overcome enormous pain....or perhaps they already had a clue...do you think?

Later, in her introduction to the aromatherapy book *Awaken to Healing Fragrance: The Power of Essential Oil Therapy by*

Elizabeth Jones, Pert explains how much more attractive plant essences are for healing than traditional medicine since they absorb so gently into the fats of the body that they do not leave residues in the liver before leaving it.

Aromatherapy then is uniquely placed to heal. On a physical level the oils bond to receptors, triggering processes leaving no toxicity behind to injure the body at a later date. On an emotional level, it addresses feelings and mindsets keeping us in unhealthy ruts, changing emotions and flooding the body with far healthier thoughts, which in turn promote better health.

Emotions and The Organs

To a healer, this correlation between the locations of the chakras and these hotspots of neuropeptides is mind blowing. But as you delve even further into the ancient philosophies you find that the ramifications are even bigger than we thought.

Chinese Medicine, in particular, offers great insights into how the emotions affect the organs. In fact, in terms of releasing and balancing emotions, I suspect acupuncture probably has the highest success rate on this particular juncture of the triangle.

Their branch of alternative medicine closely aligns the organs with seven specific emotions that pass through the body. These are:

- Anger

- Fear

- Fright

- Grief

- Joy

- Worry and Pensiveness

Notice how similar this list is to Plutchik's Primary Emotions.

It is believed that the body is always in a state of flux of the emotions. Some days we will be more joyous than others, and some days more frightened too. In the same way, there will be days when it is less so.

It is agreed that balance is the key component in health and whilst every emotion is healthy, there are times when the emotion can become too severe or too mild. This then, is when the organs are bought into play. TCM speaks of the importance of qi (Chi), the vital life force running through our bodies, keeping us healthy, vibrant and well.

Clearly, all emotions, in balance are healthy, useful and should be expressed. Health problems occur when the [body]mind lingers too long on one prevailing emotion. Then, organic imbalance begins to take place.

The corresponding emotions and their organs are: Anger affects the liver, fear and fright lodges in the kidneys, grief suffocates the lungs, joy warms the heart, worry and pensiveness unbalance the spleen. Let's look at those in more detail.

Liver

Corresponding emotion: Anger

This aspect is covered in far more detail in the Essential Oil Liver Cleanse, where we examine the emotional elements very deeply. But here, suffice it to say: anger has many guises and varying degrees, not least rage, resentment and frustration.

For a moment, try those labels on for size. As you imagine up feeling rage, can you feel how it has a very different physical vibration from resentment. Perhaps it even creates a different facial expression? One would presume we will soon find different peptides are at play. Each is an expression of anger, but a different shade and circumstance.

Anger has a wood element, so is inflammatory. It causes the qi of the body to ascend, and we can get this wooziness we associate with heights

- Vertex Headache

- Dizziness

- Blurry Vision

- Blood Pressure is Raised

- Stroke

- Inability to make decisions (I'm so angry, I can't think straight)

Because grief is a metal element, we say it controls the wood of anger. Cutting though it and, of course, numbing it.

Gall bladder

Corresponding emotion: Pent up and anger and frustration. It is also affected by people bottling up emotions.

This organ is most affected when there is a diet of greasy, fatty foods. It is also found to be troublesome when it has to deal with hot damp environments.

Which came first then? The anger and the need to comfort eat pie and chips? Or did the food make the person angry? That, my dear reader...is the six million dollar question! But there is always this strange correlation where you will see the emotion and the physical aspect working together.

On the physical level, gall bladder imbalance also affects hormones, in particular the ovaries and the thyroid, as well as obesity. So.... Polycystic ovarian syndrome...overweight and ovaries playing up.....

Incidentally the gall bladder and the liver always affect each other, too, because the organs work in pairs.

There can also be an increase in food sensitivities and a persistently runny nose. (Those of you who go onto read the Aromatherapy Eczema Treatment, will smile when you see what an effects of non alcoholic fatty liver disease has on allergies).

Kidneys

Corresponding element: Fear and fear

The kidneys house the constitution we inherited from our parents. On a physical level, whether you are a strong and resiliently healthy person or a sickly creature. On an emotional level, were you encouraged to take on the world on or to shrink away from it to safety.

Fear makes Qi descend and so we have this idea that vibrancy is being forced down. And, indeed, we see concentration being compromised because thinking controls fear, but conversely fear also begins to overwhelm the thoughts.

For my own part, when dad was dying, my prevailing fear was that I couldn't face the world without him. He had always been my defender and my crutch and I was terrified I was not strong enough to fight my own battles alone. Fear, kidneys, parents.....

Low kidney energy can make you feel lonely and insecure; vitality then becomes compromised. An interesting paradox is that fear also has a huge effect on urinary control. A person can wet themselves because they are frightened (adults but of course, scared little kids too.) In 2015 I am releasing a book about Chronic Pelvic Pain Syndrome. One of the symptoms of this is urinary incontinence coupled with urinary retention: the mind controls it, entirely through perceived fear.

On the surface, fear and fright may seem very closely aligned. But fright is a very sudden thing and pertains to something that happened in the past. Fear, by opposition is chronic, growing, lingering over a long period of time and relates to a perceived threat that the future might offer. Think then, of the child who has been perpetually abused. That repeated fright turns into a fear of what can happen in the future.

Again, don't forget the triangle mind...body...spirit. The kidneys can make you feel lonely...or maybe the loneliness affects the kidneys.

Earlier you read the soldier's account of fear, and he spoke of the smell of sweat changing in fear. PTSD patients excrete far higher levels of dopamine in their urine. This is the hormone connected with fear and is not only found in the brain but is synthesised in the kidneys.

An imbalance in kidney energy also harms the Liver and Gallbladder

You can expect to see symptoms such as

- Depression

- Indecision

- Confusion

- Lacking in Courage

- Aggression

- Anxiety, restlessness

Heart
Corresponding Emotion: Joy
Chakra - Heart

It is easy as a Westerner to picture what a deficiency of joy might look like (there is a telling statement on our quality of life, if ever there was one) but an excess of joy is harder. This might be because of a discrepancy in translation in ancient texts. The excess of joy is pronounced xi which can mean *over excited* or *over eating*. We all know what over eating will ultimately do to the heart. In the same way imagine getting some amazingly joyous news that makes you cry, and that causes a headache; excess of joy!

Joy slows the journey of qi through the body. I find it helpful to draw a parallel with the physical body and circulation, the blood is pumped around the body by the heart. The happier a person is, the likelier they are to enjoy lower blood pressure.

Joy is a fire element (she has a real fire in her belly). In the same way fire is controlled by water, then fear (which has a water element) controls joy. Consider too, what fear does to the circulation. It drives up blood pressure, and of course a person without a worry in the world is likely to enjoy far lower pressure.

When joy edges past balance and into the realms of a bi-polar extreme, again we have this fury, speedy, manic edge. Life seems to be, very much, in the fast lane.

The physical presentation of this OTT joy energy is likely to show itself as:

Palpitations, Insomnia, Unclear Thinking, Mania, Risk-Taking and Heart Attack.

73

Spleen

Corresponding emotion: Worry and pensiveness

Chakra- Solar Plexus

The body's thoughts and intentions are housed in the spleen. I often find it interesting that some sources align it to worry, others to pensiveness and again, this seems to have the same idea as the kidney. Worry about something: looking forward. Pensiveness, it seems to me, is a more melancholy nostalgia, looking back.

In balance, we find intelligence and ideas. Out of kilter we have frustration and explosive anger – consider the parallel "Vent your spleen".

According to Chinese Medicine, the spleen directs memories, sending them to the kidney in the short term and heart over the long term.

The positive emotions connected with the spleen are trust, openness and impartiality. Negative ones are worry, obsessiveness, obsessions, remorse, regret and self doubt. Regular readers of my books will know I have three beautiful children. The middle child has Asperger's Syndrome, and so this parallel with obsessions set me on a trail of research. I have since found that indeed, balancing the spleen is recommended in the treatment of Autistic Spectrum children! It is also connected to memory, focus and study.

Stomach

Corresponding emotion – worry

Chakra – Solar Plexus

The spleen is paired with the stomach which also becomes absolutely fascinating, when you discover scientists now agree we actually have two completely separate nervous systems. Surrounding the stomach is, what is called, the *Enteric Nervous System*. A massive hundred million neurons are involved in its activity, making it as complex as the spinal column. Often, it is referred to as "The Second Brain".

In a healthy body, this would normally communicate with the brain through the parasympathetic nervous system (the vagus nerve), but studies now show that if the nerve is severed, this Second Brain is able to work completely independently, with no input from the central nervous system, carrying messages about peristalsis, digestion etc.

Now, what do you remember about the location of scrotonin in the body? 90% of the body's "happiness" neuropeptides, are found, not in the brain, but in the gut as well as 50% of the "desire/dread" peptide dopamine.

Wow! Stress affects Irritable Bowel....? I should say so!

Bowels

Corresponding Emotion – I no longer have use for this.

Chakra: solar plexus

Bowels represent that which is now surplus to our needs. Those things we want to eliminate. Clearly in the physical sense this is not just food but also the de-oxygenated red blood cells that are now defunct and lead to the colour of our faeces. But how does that relate on an emotional level?

Problems with digestion is very much solar plexus energy and can often communicate there is a problem with self expression of thoughts of emotions. They often betray how we are trying to control life rather than going with the flow.

You might recognise the notion of a rumbling appendix which on closer examination might reveal an extreme emotion that literally growls, pushed down and suppressed rather than let go after it had served its purpose.

For a person who has problems letting go of emotions, belongings or even knowledge, you might find them also holding on too tightly to their stools, for constipation. What's more the person may also feel life is no longer nourishing them, it perhaps has gone stale.

Diarrhoea by direct contrast often emanates from the inability to achieve your goals or get what you want. This idea of things running away from you...or perhaps, never managing to reach the finish line comes to mind. This can be made even worse by the fact people suffering from this energy keep on facing similar life lessons over and over again and yet are failing to learn and absorb them. Often empowering a patient using oils such as rosewood to focus their concentration of frankincense to improve their confidence can regulate the bowels.

Irritable Bowel Syndrome is a fascinating conflict of the two. Consider that the person may be afraid of asking for what they want from life and so they keep hold back from asking.

Lungs

Corresponding Emotion: *Grief*

Chakra: Heart

This connection is best understood in two ways. The first is through sobbing. This wailing element, as one cries at one's loss, means you take in massive gulps of air. The second way is to understand is to consider the notion that taking in air is one's way of nourishing the body. Clearly, this is with oxygen, but also new ideas, vital flow of love.

If a person does not express their grief honestly and properly, then this nourishment does not have a chance to find its way into their system. They are stuck and do not move on. They stagnate in a circumstance that no longer has a future.

Lung energy can often become depressed because a person has expended all of their energy on a person, (or thing) outside of themselves for a long period, leading to their own nourishment not being fulfilled. Naturally this would certainly apply to nursing a loved one in their last days, for instance. When they have gone, this only leads to deeper feelings of "What next? Where do I go from here?" One does not need a Phd in complementary medicine to know a useful way forward is to help this person find a new focus, a new joy that will fulfil her again.

Conversely, just as we might find perpetual coughing and wheezing in those early days, we should look for similar emotions when a person exhibits bronchitis, pleurisy, pneumonia. Most dangerously we see manifestations of these illnesses or even lung cancers, in people who cannot find a way to let go of the past.

Some symptoms you might see manifesting with this organ/ emotion correlation are:

- Tightness in the Chest (Shortness of breath)

- Excessive Crying

- Asthma

- Frequent Colds and Flu

- Skin problems

- Grief Affecting the Heart

- Circulation issues

Some more interesting emotional/ physical correlations:

Skin

Corresponding emotion – low self esteem

Chakra - Crown

Our skin represents our perception of how the world sees us, that outer persona we extend to others. Often issues concerning the skin belie dissatisfaction about how we see ourselves. In my book The Aromatherapy Eczema Treatment we investigate how the feelings of imperfection and frustration can spiral into an enraged episode of scratching. Similar mindsets often underlie acne and psoriasis too.

Genitals

Corresponding emotion: I feel safe in my sexuality

Chakra: Sacral

There is a direct relationship about how we feel about our sexuality and how our body manifests this. The emotion seems best described as being "how we feel about giving and receiving love". Do we feel strong in our femininity/masculinity? Indeed do we feel safe to express it, and confident we will receive a welcoming response in return?

Blood

Corresponding Emotion: I don't feel good about this

Chakra: Crown and Heart

When there are issues with circulation and the blood, perhaps the body is communicating you do not feel at one with yourself over something. It often betrays weak internal foundations. Often there are reasons you feel you cannot connect to what is happening in your own physicality. With blood disorders it is not uncommon to discover the sufferer no longer has a sense of love pulsating in their lives.

Immunity

Corresponding Emotion: I am, what I am!

Chakra: Heart

Conflict over being able to *be what you want* and *have what you want*. The most extreme example of this is HIV, which of course, is an elegant metaphor for the challenges of the homosexual community in the '8os. How strange that the advancements in medication that would come to help suffers of this illness should co-incide with a freer, more open and accepting opinion about homosexuality. Could this openness have allowed these people to strengthen their own immunity without even having any insights into the correlation?

Peak Flow of Organs

Just for reference, because it is interesting to plot when systemic patterns seem at their most troublesome...there is a cycle of peak flow of each of the organs.

Lung	3 to 5 am	Peak 4 am
Large Intestine	5 to 7 am	Peak 6 am
Stomach	7 to 9 am	Peak 8 am
Spleen	9 to 11 am	Peak 10 am
Heart	11 to 1 pm	Peak 12 pm
Small Intestine	1 to 3 pm	Peak 2 pm
Urinary Bladder	3 to 5 pm	Peak 4 pm
Kidney	5 to 7 pm	Peak 6 pm
Pericardium	7 to 9 pm	Peak 8 am
Triple Warmer	9 to 11 pm	Peak 10 pm

Gall Bladder	11 to 1 am	Peak 12 am
Liver	1 to 3 am	Peak 2 am

Part 2 - The Holistic Principle

The kind of medicine I deal in is Complementary Medicine. I use that term instead of the *Alternative* Medicine which some of you may be more familiar with. There are two reasons for this.

The first is this. I have been a practitioner for over 20 years, but I trained for just two. Physicians, GPs whatever your country refers to them as, could wipe the floor with my knowledge. They are the experts on how the body works. If a doctor gives my patients medicine to take...I insist they take it. My medicine works complementary to theirs.

The second reason is, in my experience often essential oils can't do the entire healing job alone. I might need to refer a patient to a chiropractor to straighten her spine for really great healing to happen. The oils might unlock memories and thoughts a counsellor is better equipped to handle. Vitamin therapy often plays a part in nourishing the body back to health. The therapies all work complementary to one another.

Above all things, the most important aspect of complementary medicine is to achieve a state of balance. For the hormones, this will be enough power to make the body tick, but not too much to create a surge. Balance might also refer to *postural* balance, in particular to the shoulders and hips and so often, a visit to the chiropractor might be suggested. Usually with stress patients, it refers to life balance. That could be balancing the hours you do at work, but also learning to allow your own wants and needs into the family mix. Often it is very counter intuitive for a patient to start thinking "what's right for me?"

Mind Body Spirit Principle

The holistic principle, very much takes its lead from the ancient healing technique of Ayurveda which says that we are made up of three separate but connected parts. These are the outer body, the inner body and the secret aspect.

The outer body is easy for us to understand. It's what you see on the outside, the hair, the bones, the teeth and the skin. The inner body too, to a certain extent is simple. The skeleton, the internal digestive and other processes, but also all the thoughts which run through the brain make up this inner part.

When the outer body and the inner body are in accord, then the shining aspect radiates through. In other philosophies we call this the spirit.

The Spirit

So what actually *is* the spirit? Quite simply it is this...the part that is quintessentially *you.* Your core values, your innate ideals, your slightly strange talents, your loves and your loathings.

Like a finger print, you are unique in this world.

So the core aspect of healing through complementary medicine is to get the person to a place where they can be who they *want* to be. They can achieve a balance where they are happy in their life, they are channelling their hopes and dreams and their body is lovin' them for it.

This.....*this,* is how we perceive wellness.

What this also means then, is there is a need from a therapeutic point of view to treat the patient in terms of their mind, their body, and their spirit.

This is to say: we treat the person, rather than their symptoms.

Funnily enough, I was speaking to one of my friends recently about the changes one seems to go through when you hit your forties. Not necessarily a midlife crisis, per se, but somehow I found (I am 43) that somehow priorities seem to have shifted and I am not longer chasing the same dreams I once was. Children changed them, my health changed them, actually nearly having my home repossessed when my husband and I were both made redundant changed them...suddenly money doesn't seem so important after all.

So why then, did I spend every waking hour worrying about what the banks wanted from me? To me, looking back, this was my spiritual crisis...but also my awakening.

The day I waved my old house goodbye, was the day I let go.

The next day I met a person I really liked very much. That person was *me*, and do you know, I don't think I had met this woman before?

Without the restraints of having to worry about the bank manager, a more creative, more self assured me started to emerge. I am certainly (internally) a quieter person than I once was. Not so angry, but also not so easily pushed about. The funny thing was, I also found I was healthier and stronger than I ever had been before.

The universe in her wisdom, had sent me a new friend, and I was helping her with some delicious empowerment articles. On the other side of the planet Luanne Simmons opened a door to a whole new me, without having a clue she had done it. Luanne's business "Goddess on Purpose" required me to consider why on earth I had been put on this earth.

A deep question, but since I had moved from the city to a tumbledown cottage, I didn't really have much else to do but sit and write in front of the fire. No friends yet, no distractions, just me, the fire and my thoughts....

They tumbled out.

When I considered the natural talents I had been born with, and the things I loved to do, I realised I was as unique as my fingerprints and there were things happening around me I had the power to change.

Thing was I had no idea what they were or what it was I was supposed to do. I sensed it, but I couldn't quite put my finger on it. But I trusted that the answer would reveal itself and I suspected when that it did, it would be like a bolt from the blue. In the meantime I gathered up my scattered skills and worked them till my fingers were sore. I improved my writing, I learned more about marketing, music and dance were levered back into my life and I waited for this thunderbolt to come.

When it did, it hit me so hard I was almost forced through the floor.

The answer was staring me in the face but I couldn't see it. I could show people how aromatherapy is so much more remarkable than they think and I could teach therapists how to take it to the forefront of medicine.

Big.

Yet, entirely within my skillset, and everything I have ever learned in my life added up to that moment.

Small...well yes, it's just writing books really isn't it?

But the most powerful thing is, I absolutely know where I am going with this. I get up in a morning and know what I am trying to achieve. I won't say I am tireless (because frankly I am knackered after writing six books in 7 months) but I am unstoppable! Because, I know where the end of the journey is for me.

So the question is, do you know where *you* are going? Do you *know* what makes you happy? Do you do enough of that...in fact do you do *any* of it?

This is the equation that starts to tie the healing together.

Get the serotonin rushing and to do that identify what it is that makes you happy.

Easy on paper, right?

Give Me Joy In My Heart...

So how does one find one's joy?

Before we start this journey, I want you to do a small exercise. It is easy to do, but I want you to put as much thought and effort into it as you can because it will reap rewards at the end.

Try to think back to the person you were when you were 9.

What were you like?

What were your hopes and dreams?

How did you feel about school?

Describe the picture you had of your mother.

What about the one you had of your father

What were your hobbies?

What interested you?

Who were your best friends?

Who did you admire?

What job would you have liked to have done?

When you imagined moving away from home, how did you imagine your free time to be?

It is a widely held belief that when we do not have rules and obligations to fulfil then our true passions shine through. As a child I would dance for hours and drive my mum insane singing hymns. Now as an adult, the same applies, I never feel truly free until there is a beat and I am swinging my hips. As for the hymns...to my mind a bit of Aled Jones never did anyone any harm.

Ok, now compare that list to your life now. In what ways have you changed, and how are you similar? Are you still running your life based on the scripts of a nine year old? I wonder? We know emotional habit and thought processes are hard to break. Are you still chasing the dreams that pre-pubescent had about financial success, when you now love money can't buy happiness, it can only rent it? Those hobbies you were doing when you had no priorities and responsibilities getting in the way, when was the last time you enjoyed those? Let's be honest, as a child you had a whole better handle on a sense of pure joy than you do now, I'll bet?

The second that the phrase "But I don't have the time" comes into your mind, remind yourself...there is a heart attack at stake.

Perhaps, even pin this poem, written by **Erma Bombeck** when she had discovered she was dying of cancer, to your fridge!

IF I HAD MY LIFE TO LIVE OVER
I would have gone to bed when I was sick instead of
pretending the earth would go into a holding pattern if I

weren't there for the day.

I would have burned the pink candle sculpted like a rose before it melted in storage.

I would have talked less and listened more.

I would have invited friends over to dinner even if the carpet was stained, or the sofa faded.

I would have eaten the popcorn in the 'good' living room and worried much less about the dirt when someone wanted to light a fire in the fireplace.

I would have taken the time to listen to my grandfather ramble about his youth.

I would have shared more of the responsibility carried by my husband.

I would never have insisted the car windows be rolled up on a summer day because my hair had just been teased and sprayed.

I would have sat on the lawn with my grass stains.

I would have cried and laughed less while watching television and more while watching life.

I would never have bought anything just because it was practical, wouldn't show soil, or was guaranteed to last a lifetime.

Instead of wishing away nine months of pregnancy, I'd have cherished every moment and realized that the wonderment growing inside me was the only chance in life to assist God in a miracle.

When my kids kissed me impetuously, I would never have said, 'Later. Now go get washed up for dinner.' There would have been more 'I love you's;' More 'I'm sorry's.'

But mostly, given another shot at life, I would seize every minute, look at it and really see it ... live it and never give it back.

So the question must be? If these thoughts are spiritual, the how do we define our spirit?

This is the part that is quintessentially you.

Your hopes, dreams, your values, talents, innate abilities, your loves and hates. I suppose it is the part of you, you cannot hide from when you close your eyes and go to sleep. It is the driving force that not only separates you from the crowd, but also guides your moral compass of what you perceive to be right or wrong.

The problem is, it very soon gets lost beneath pay checks and piles of washing. (Look in the knicker drawer, under that leopard skin thong, you might see a sparkle of spirit under there!)

But how do we start to build these parts of our spirit back into our lives? Certainly those childhood joys are believed to hold a key.

My mum, Jill Bruce, loved to play with her pattern bricks exploring colours and geometry. How strange that today she is the author of **The Aura and Out of The Labyrinth,** a book that investigates the part sacred geometry plays in healing depression.

Anna Goodwin is an accountant. For many years, she was puzzled by this exercise because the only love she could really identify was her coloured pencils and pad. It perplexed her how on earth that could match up with the job she had chosen for herself. Now as an adult, she has used this passion to make workbooks which help new businesses navigate the joys of tax returns and bank reconciliations. Each booklet has lovely pictures of Alan and Bert, a vexed painter and decorator and his, extremely helpful accountant who take the reader step by step through how to do the accounts and what pieces of paper you do and don't need.

What made me laugh was for weeks when she had a bad day at work, she would say she was taking herself off to the sofa to work on her books. On the occasional days when she could not find joy at work she *channelled* it playing with blues, greens and reds. And of course in channelling her passion, she has not only made herself happier but she can help millions of account-shy businesses start to smile too. If you think these might be useful to you, you can find her details at **buildyourownreality.com/anna-goodwin/**

Of course, not all of our passions stay the same as when we were children, we discover new ones too. If I don't get much work done in a day, it can usually be blamed on the same culprits, scruffy, fluffy, darling baby birds whom I love watching exploring my bird table....or possibly you might find me making a cake.

Interestingly though, the birds discovery came from simply sitting quietly, away from the stress of work, when I slowed down enough to notice what was happening so very close by.

And the circle continues, slow down, learn, slow down and learn some more.

Somehow, it seems to me that Caroline Myss is entirely correct in her *Anatomy of The Spirit*, that wellness comes when you start to detach from seeing success as a goal...but rather as an energy of self control. Paying attention to our thoughts and feelings, and focusing on the intention of being calmer, happier and more flexible in our attitudes seems to be key.

What I will say at this point is clinical healing is my realm. There are far better spiritual advisors than I. For your own development in understanding the spiritual nuances and healing potential of essential oils I cannot recommend Jill Bruce's Garden of Eden enough. From the other side of the coin (and actually your own exploration of spirit) Angela Mckay's Wise Woman's Journal are a fascinating journey into contemplations of spiritual thoughts and vibrations each day. It is beautiful, but grounded and sensible in a rather effervescent way. You can download a complimentary past edition of this at **buildyourownreality.com/wwj-back-copy/**

Part 3 The Healing

Meditation

Every one of the sources I have cited in this book are united in the belief that the single most effective way to quieten the mind and lift your vibration is through meditation. Research shows that people who practice regularly have a slower, healthier and more focused resting brain wave. This means their concentration is better; they are more relaxed and in turn more healthy too.

There are many ways to meditate, but for the purposes of this book we shall focus on vitalising and balancing the chakras.

You will often see people meditating sitting in the lotus position, so they have contact with the root chakra and the floor. It is not necessary to sit cross legged, you can achieve the same objective sitting upright in a chair or lying on your back on the bed.

Close your eyes and breathe slowly and deliberately. We want to build the breathing up in cycles where we breathe in for four and out for eight. This is the cycle used in transcendental meditation and has been proven to be the best way to release endorphins in the brain, which of course is useful for pain relief.

Once you have mastered the breathing pattern, see a white light coming out of your head, like a fountain and coming down the side of your body, completely surrounding it. Let the light do this six times so you are entirely surrounded and completely protected by it. We call this psychically protecting ourselves. This is vital and you must do this every time you meditate (and every time you heal or massage someone).

Now we are going to focus on the chakras and we want to see them start to pulsate open and closed, regularly, rhythmically and brightly.

At the brow see a violet light above your head.

Then when you are happy it is bright and energetic, move your focus to the brow and visualise a deep rich indigo there.

At the throat, see blue.

The heart, green.

Yellow at the solar plexus

Orange at the abdomen

Red at the root.

Then when you are happy they are nourished and vital, repeat the white light fountain six more complete times around you.

Lastly imagine a beautiful golden rain, cleansing your white bubble washing away any germs impurities or negative energy you may have collected.

Open your eyes.

That really was the dummies guide!!! There is far more information in **Out of the Labyrinth**, focusing on how to gain insights and healing whilst in meditation. I also like to use chakra singing bowl recordings off youtube because I am a more auditory person and find that method simpler.

Hypnosis

For me, I find hypnosis is easier and more effective, but that is simply personal choice. If you would like to try some hypnotherapy relaxation (for free) please feel free to download an MP3 made by my very good friend Mark of Mark Bowden Hypnotherapy who has made this download especially for readers of my books. You can find it at *buildyourownreality.com/free-hypnosis-download/*

Essential oils for chakra healing

Some oils which vibrate on the chakras are:

Crown

Frankincense, Palma Rosa, Cumin, Sandalwood,

Brow

Aniseed, Camomile Roman, Cardamom, Clary Sage, Hop,

Jasmine, Camomile Maroc, Carrot, Rose Geranium, Tea Tree, Valerian, Rose Otto (Enfleurage),

Throat

Cypress, Dill, Ginger, Bulgarian Lavender, Rose Otto (Distilled) Peppermint, Neroli

Heart

Amber, Basil, Bay, Benzoin, Lavandin, Mandarin, Orange, Spearmint, Rose Maroc, Rose geranium,

Cajuput, Lavender, Peppermint, Neroli

Solar Plexus

Cade, Cajuput, Cedarwood, Cypress, Dill, Garlic, Ginger, Grapefruit, Helichrysm, Oregano, Rosemary, Bulgarian Lavender, Rose Otto (Distilled) Peppermint, Neroli

Sacral

Black Pepper, Tonka Bean, Peppermint, Rose Otto Distillation

Base or root

Clove

For a more in depth understanding of how the oils will affect the chakras and the etheric bodies of the aura, please see: **Jill Bruce's Garden of Eden.** There are dozens more oils for you to choose from there.

The Emotions

The theory of the eight primary emotions has been expanded and developed over recent years. The full list of primary emotions is known to be:

- Joy

- Happiness

- Satisfaction

- Fulfilment

- Contentment

- Peace

- Fear

- Shame

- Sadness

- Hurt

- Guilt

- Frustration

- Dissatisfaction

- Disappointment

The discerning eye will notice this is a mixed list of positive and negative emotions. Psychiatrists agree there is no such thing as a feeling that should not be expressed, rather ones that ought not be acted upon. Each emotion has value, it teaches us things about our own responses and ordeals and it will affect the way we think in the future.

Primary emotions are the ones that happen immediately in a scenario, and are, for the most part, fleeting and transient. In some instances we will respond automatically. For instance, our sudden fear ensures we jump out of the way of an oncoming car. The action is so fast that our body reacts unconsciously. For a large proportion of time though our inner voice niggles at us telling us what we should and should not think and the expression of these primary emotions begins to change. Over time, primary emotions that have not been effectively expressed will gradually merge into secondary emotions.

These are:

- Disapproval

- Disdain

- Hatred

- Coldness

- Hostility

- Persecution Complex

- Paranoia

- Distrust

- Jealousy

- Worry

- Anxiety

- Insecurity

- Low Self Esteem

- Self-hatred

- Depression

- Anger/Rage

For the most part it is these stagnant and festering emotions that pollute our systems, preventing the easy flow of energy and causing illness to erupt.

So at this point, we might consider how we can make this intervention into our emotions/health situation, and the answer is most certainly by paying close attention to our thought patterns...

And then intentionally changing them.

With practice it becomes very easy to recognise when you are being influenced by some kind of fear pattern and to start to exert some control over the situation.

The key is to be able to isolate the emotions in terms of some kind of time scale. Remember:

Primary emotions are the initial emotions during and just after an event. But then, within minutes these can start to morph into secondary emotions which can mask the initial response and so they can make it harder to isolate the true emotion at play which is hidden deeper beneath the secondary feelings. Just to make things more complicated, Plutchik also believed there were tertiary emotions. These secondary emotions and thoughts which reinforce them ensure the body is subjected over and over, to floods of the corresponding neurotransmitters. The body mind becomes addicted to them, ensuring you keep replenishing their stocks to the tissues of the body. It is no wonder then, we develop strong habits of thinking from a very early age.

It is important then, to really try (perhaps during meditation) to centre the emotions and also to contemplate what the fundamental emotions are that are causing stress in your life.

From here, we can start to recommend some oils to start to move the emotions on to a healthier place.

So for example if the resounding emotion seems to be humiliation, we can see the secondary response was most likely to have been shame. The underlying primary one though, is sadness.

I have listed oils for the foundation primary emotion, there are secondary and tertiary emotions listed below to help you find the pathway back to the source. There are oils for the primary emotions, some for the secondary and tertiary, but I have not been able to cover them all (yet) but it is a very comprehensive list. Interestingly, although much is taken from Worwood's

Fragrant Mind and *Aromantics,* most of the correlations come from Jill Bruce's Garden of Eden.

I have not added methods of application as this is covered in the free resource *The Complete Guide to Clinical Aromatherapy and Essential Oils for The Physical Body.* To my mind, diffusers and evaporators work very well and of course integrating these oils into massage will have marvellous effects.

One possible thought is that if Patricia Davis asserts that oils used in larger concentrations lift the benefits of the physical realm and into the emotional and spiritual, so you might want to experiment with slightly stronger dilutions of some of the safer oils, seven or even ten drops in a blend.

There are some strong oils here, also some contraindications (shown with * and are listed at the end of the passage). You might want to go for homeopathic doses of these, for example, I would not thank you for massaging me with garlic....

Anger

To quell anger - *Ylang Ylang* - regains balance and perspective; helps to "let go".

The **Secondary emotions** of **Anger** are:

Irritation, exasperation, rage, disgust, envy, torment.

Exploring those in more depth:

Irritation

Its tertiary emotions are:

Aggravation, irritation, agitation, annoyance, grouchiness, grumpiness

For someone who seems riddled with annoyance – *Camomile*

If they seem easily irritated and irascible – *Sandalwood*

Exasperation

Its tertiary emotion is : Frustration

- Ease frustration - *Anise**, helps you to bide your time

- *Citronella* - helps ideas flow,

- *Niaoulli*-breeds patience

- *Jasmine* -sexual problems and frustration

- *Marjoram* for enforced celibacy

Rage

Its tertiary emotions are:

outrage, fury, wrath, hostility, ferocity, bitterness, hate, scorn, spite, vengefulness, dislike, resentment

Sage*- takes the edge off fierce violent rage.

Rosemary* - Dissipates the drive for revenge

Tangerine* - Cuts through spite

Cade – Again, spite

Disgust

Its tertiary emotions are:

Revulsion, contempt, loathing

Suffering disgust (closed mental doors) - *Violet Leaf* - Opens areas of the mind that have been closed

Envy

Its tertiary emotions are:

Revulsion, contempt, loathing, jealousy

Curb envy - *Tangerine*- cuts through spite

Ylang Ylang - dissipates jealousy

Torment

There are no tertiary emotions

Valerian – Helps a person hide from their problems temporarily

Camomile Maroc- shrink under problems

Rose Otto – Serene calm

Sadness
Primary emotion

Top of the list is *bergamot*.

*The **secondary emotions** of sadness are:*

Suffering, sadness, disappointment, shame, neglect, despair

Exploring these in more detail...

Suffering

Its tertiary emotions are:

Agony, suffering, hurt, anguish

Bergamot - Hurt

Sadness

Its tertiary emotions are:

Depression, despair, hopelessness, gloom, glumness, sadness, unhappiness, grief, sorrow, woe, misery, melancholy

Remove despair - *Benzoin* is a liberating oil

Hope - *Citronella*

Come to terms with grief – *Rose*

Angelica- understands death

Disappointment

Its tertiary emotions are:

Dismay, disappointment, displeasure

Disappointment -*Patchouli*

Shame

Its tertiary emotions are:

Guilt, shame, regret, remorse, neglect, alienation, isolation, neglect, loneliness, rejection, homesickness, defeat, dejection, insecurity, embarrassment, humiliation, insult

Embarrassment – *Jasmine* – sexual

Spearmint- of incidents in the past

Reduce guilt - *Camphor** -esp. religious guilt.

Clove for those who have to race around in life and miss their children

Rose de mai -love affairs

Alleviate shame - *Oakmoss Resin*- helps lift traumas of the past

Vertivert - deep hidden secrets.

Sympathy

Its tertiary emotions are:

Pity, sympathy

Fear

Primary Emotion

The **Secondary Emotions** of **Fear** are: ***Horror, nervousness***

Exploring these in more detail:

Horror

Its tertiary emotions are:

Alarm, shock, fear, fright, horror, terror, panic, hysteria, mortification

Amber – Lifts trauma

Oakmoss Resin – Brings negative memories to the fore.

Angelica - understands death

Incidentally, I am not going to explain the mechanisms of saying **PTSD** and *celery seed*, because they form a large part of The Professional Stress Solution, but yes...*celery seed* because it helps with oxytocin and bonding mechanisms.

Shock - *Camphor*, Valerian*

Nervousness

Its tertiary emotions are:

Anxiety, nervousness, tenseness, uneasiness, apprehension, worry, distress, dread

Nervousness: *Violet Leaf, Camomile, Geranium*

Apprehension - *Valerian, Camphor**- fear of others hurting them

Make decisions to change and stick with them - *Rosemary*

Helplessness - *Coriander* - Courage to press ahead; follow through with decision

Powerlessness - *Frankincense*- Confidence

Worry - *Geranium* interfaces mental and emotional. Especially helps financial worry.

Cedarwood -clears unwanted thoughts

Dispel doubt - *Frankincense* instils confidence

Birch- helps see the truth of a situation

Self worth – *Thyme, Jasmine*

Trust

Calendula - confidence that you can make the right decision

Stress - *Lavender, Camomile, Geranium*

Tension – *Geranium*

Love
Primary Emotion

Oils to inspire love: *Rose, jasmine, agarwood*

The **secondary** emotions of **love** are: **Affection, lust, longing**

Exploring those in more detail:

Affection

Its tertiary emotions are:

Adoration, liking, attraction, caring, tenderness, compassion, sentimentality

Affection – *lavender, cypress*

Fondness - *patchouli*

Caring – *Lavender (Bulgarian), Lavender (English), Camomile maroc*

Tenderness - *Mimosa*

Compassion – *Spearmint*

Harmony in the home - *Mimosa*

Joy of motherhood- *Celery Seed* - helps motherhood bonding

Lust

Its tertiary emotions are:

Arousal, desire, lust, passion, infatuation

Arounsal: *Jasmine, ylang ylang, patchouli, sandalwood, agarwood, tuberose*

(also if there is a need to curb the lust or infatuation for some reason – marjoram)

Longing

No tertiary emotions.

Marjoram to curb sexual longing.

Joy

Primary Emotion

Bergamot is top of the list but any of your predominately aldehydic oils:

Melissa, lemon verbena, citronella, lemon.

The secondary emotions of joy are: Cheerfulness, zest, contentment, pride, optimism, enthrallment, relief

Cheerfulness

Its tertiary emotions are:

Amusement, bliss, cheerfulness, gaiety, glee, jolliness, joviality, joy, delight, enjoyment, gladness, happiness, jubilation, elation, satisfaction, ecstasy, euphoria

Amusement - *Mandarin-* creates a partylike atmosphere

Delight - *Palmarosa-* gentle happiness

Zest

Its tertiary emotions are:

Enthusiasm, zeal, zest, excitement, thrill, exhilaration

Elation - *Clary Sage-* (be careful not to over use.)

Excitement - *Lemon-* uplifting

Contentment

Its tertiary emotions are:

Contentment, pleasure

Calm - *Camomile maroc*

Contentment - *Caraway*- at peace with life,

Agarwood – satisfaction with one's lot in life.

Silver Fir- happiness to "just be"

Thyme - content with your lot

Relaxation - *Lavender, Geranium, Jasmine*

Happiness - *Orange*

Hyacinth - childlike lightness; able to see the joy in life

Cardamom – feeling a comfortable life

Pride

Its tertiary emotions are:

Pride, triumph

Orange – Seeing what you are capable of

Thyme – Feeling happy with one's place in life

Optimism

Its tertiary emotions are:

Eagerness, hope, optimism

Citronella - Hope

Enthrallment

Its tertiary emotions are:

Enthrallment, rapture

Tackle boredom - *Garlic* - helps take mediocrity of life in one's stride

Interest - *Fennel*- overcomes boredom, brings perseverance & motivation

Relief

No tertiary.

Relief - *Geranium*- lets cares lift away, weight off your shoulders,

Serenity - *Caraway* - helps day ebb away

Surprise

Its tertiary emotions are:

Amazement, surprise, astonishment

No suggested oils

Contraindications of this section

Please refer to The Complete Guide for Clinical Aromatherapy and Essential Oils for the Physical Body for full safety data on specific oils. This is available as a free resource on many book platforms.

However, please do not use any essential oils in the first 16 weeks of pregnancy.

Sage* promotes heavy bleeding in women and so use 1/15th of a drop only

Rosemary – neurotoxic contraindicated in epilepsy or schizophrenia

Conclusion

Well, there isn't really a conclusion here is there? Because this is just the start....

And here's where it starts to get interesting.

We understand two main factors are making us ill. The first is environmental toxicity, the second is our general demeanour. Whilst we can't do anything about genetics, we certainly can do plenty relax ourselves and feel a bit happier too.

Baby steps, isn't that what they say.

For the first part of the equation, dealing with toxicity, my work is done. Book three explains this cataclysmic onslaught of poisons we are subjecting our bodies too, and how to harness the natural abilities of your body to cleanse itself. Not surprisingly aromatherapy is a wonderful tool here, but also vitamins and minerals and acupressure points and diet also play a massive part.

The Professional Stress Solution wages war on that awful neuropeptide CRF1 and cortisol, and seeks to help you to understand how to bring a patient back to physical and emotional homeostasis.

Addressing the second part requires me to shut myself into the blue and green shed for a few months, because I suspect we would all like to know more about specific oils and peptides. So I am off to make some new contacts in labs, read some more clinical research and write some more notes.

Please read on through more of the books, not least the Aromatherapy Eczema Treatment because that really is emotional/physical dis-ease in practice. And of course, if you are a therapist, start writing notes in the margin of Sales Strategies for Gentle Souls about how you can implement this new knowledge into your business plan to transform your business.

As usual, I can't tell you how much it means to me that you have made your way to this page, and you have even bought the book! So thank you. Please, do remember to leave a review, won't you.

As for me...I have an appointment with 5-HT, see you soon...

Review and Buy!

Bye!

Liz

About the Author

Elizabeth Ashley qualified as an aromatherapist in 1993, and then passed her Advanced Aromatherapy Diploma in 1994. She has been practicing aromatherapy for almost 21 years.

In 1999, she fell into a whole new career in the aggressive commercial sector of recruitment consultancy. There she discovered her father's second hand car salesman genes had passed along and found she had quite a gift of the gab! More than that, she discovered she could sell...and then some.

In 2008, Elizabeth fell ill during pregnancy with a blood clot in her lungs. The pulmonary embolism prevented her from working and she started to write. Very quickly she gained her first contract as a ghost writer...a recipe book for cheese cakes!

In 2010 she was published professionally for her work on Galbanum oil in the Aromatherapy Thymes, journal of the International Federation of Aromatherapists, and on Tuberose oil by the New Zealand Register of Holistic Therapist.

In 2011 she was seconded on a consultative basis to Walsall Independent Treatment Centre, designed to be a rainbow bridge between traditional and complementary medicines. There she became aware of the rumblings of change in healthcare. Her book *Sales Strategies for Gentle Souls* explains the connotations of this.

In 2014 she ranks in the top 50 contract writers on the freelancer marketplace Elance.com. She is the ghost writer of seven number one Amazon best sellers in the natural healing category. She lives in Shropshire with her husband and youngest son, kept company by their cat, the budgie and many shoals of tropical fish! Her elder son and daughter attend University and make her prouder than anything ever could.

Elizabeth Ashley is The Secret Healer. Her books are designed to fill gaps in aromatherapy knowledge and train therapists to bring their business into the cyber age and make their practices excel.

Other Works by The Author

Book 1 - The Complete Guide to

Clinical Aromatherapy & Essential Oils for the Physical Body

Essentially...essential oils for beginners, talented novices and intermediate aromatherapists

Let me ask you, why do you want a book on aromatherapy?

Do you want to learn how to care for your family naturally?

Perhaps you have a franchise selling essential oils and want to know more about what they can do?

Maybe you love the delicious scents and want understand how these beautiful things come to heal.

I wonder if you have started to learn and now want to discover how to build on your knowledge.

Whatever you are looking for this book has something for you.

- Details of how to treat over 60 conditions with essential oils
- Profiles of over 100 natural plant essences and their safety data

- Descriptions of 15 carrier oils and their applications not only for massage but also adding to creams and lotions.
- Comprehensive data of how the chemistry of an oil will affect its actions
- In depth insights into how professional aromatherapists blend...including their 13 favourite recipes from their practices.

Including....

- Sensuous aromatherapy blends by a qualified sex therapist
- Two blends for labour by the midwife running an aromatherapy program on an NHS maternity ward
- A blend for depression by a qualified mental health

PLUS....

10 bonus essential oil monographs and a complementary hypnotherapy relaxation download.

Discount vouchers of treatments courses and products by participating therapists.

This is my gift to you.

FREE - From 30.11.14

Book 3 The Essential Oil Liver Cleanse

The Professional Aromatherapist's Liver Detox

We are warned of the threats of heart attacks, strokes and cancer, especially if we are overweight.

What is kept quieter is doctors have established a link between toxicity in the liver and metabolic syndrome, the condition that leads to many of these conditions. What's more non fatty liver disease is known to underlie many other conditions such as eczema, allergies and headaches.

The scandal is just how many of our livers are struggling under the strain of over processed foods, pharmaceutical debris and actually even our own bad tempers!

This book explains:

- The importance of the liver and its functions
- How it becomes dysfunctional and how to interpret warning signposts
- How to cleanse and nourish using not just essential oils, but also vitamins and minerals and diet.
- The strange correlation between how our emotions translate negativity into disease.

- How to implement other therapies such as chiropractic, acupressure and counselling and how to secure fantastic referrals.

This book is best used in tandem with The Professional Stress Solution to benefit from the complementary healing. Use Sales Strategies for Gentle Souls to create a marketing plan to use your new found knowledge to smash your competition out of the water!!!

Book 4 The Professional Stress Solution

Essential Oils and Holistic Health Stress Management Techniques for The Professional Aromatherapist

Stress is pandemic in our society.

Scientists agree it plays a quintessential role in how likely it is we will suffer from chronic and possibly fatal illnesses in the future. Risk factors of metabolic syndrome, diabetes, stroke and heart disease are increased through stress.

The daft thing is....aromatherapy can do amazing things to ease it, and potentially aromatherapists could take a massive workload away from the doctor's surgeries.

- Discover the hormonal changes and peptide triggers that change a person's health and mental state.
- Learn how it affects the liver, adrenals and pituitary gland.
- Uncover the strange phenomenon of Yin disease
- Build a better foundation of care, but also a knowledge base that means you can sell your treatments more effectively.
- Improve your healing skills set
- Supercharge your referrals potential from other complementary therapists and orthodox medicine alike.

Includes free bonus material of

- Chiropractic chart of misalignments and potential organic disturbance
- Chart of the meridians and suggested acupressure points to detox the organs more quickly
- Detailed information about how to improve the patients condition with vitamin and minerals therapy
- In depth dietary advice
- Free hypnotherapy relaxation download

Essential Oils are The Off Switch for stress. The *Professional Stress Solution* is the ON SWITCH for your aromatherapy business.

Book 5 The Aromatherapy Eczema Treatment

Healing Eczema, Itchy Skin Rashes and Atopic Dermatitis with Essential Oils and Holistic Medicine

Most people appreciate that the itching and redness of eczema can be used using essential oils, but what if I told you they were capable of so much more?

Imagine if, as a therapist, you were able to pinpoint the emotions that set off these flares? Can you visualise what it would mean to your patient if you were able to isolate the very protagonist causing the eczema breakout and alleviate their pain completely?

Well now you can.

This book teaches you:

- How to isolate the emotions causing the emotional cycle of pain
- The likely food triggers for your patient and the tools to identify the exact times they will detonate a reaction
- The familial traits and links that lead to atopic eczema
- How these links connect with the liver and in turn how to cleanse the liver toxicity
- Vitamins and minerals to cleanse and nourish the system

The book contains very real that will not only transform the way you treat clients, but will skyrocket your clinic's takings.

I recommend reading this book in tandem with *The Professional Stress Solution* and the *Essential Oil Liver Cleanse* to fully understand the cycles and processes of treatment. Add to it *Sales Strategies for Gentle Souls* and your business will stand on an entirely new footing.

Why not save yourself 1/3

And treat yourself to the set?

The full and comprehensive course into how to heal eczema

with aromatherapy and essential oils **$7.99 / £5.99**

I promise you...nothing else comes even close.

Sales Strategies for Gentle Souls

Targeted Sales Training for Professional Aromatherapists

Wonderful things are happening in complementary therapy. Very gifted people are churning out fantastic research and results. The internet is full of what essential oils can do. But when a gentle soul emerges from their relaxing haze of their aromatherapy class room, how do they harness the buzz of energy around them for their craft?

From 1999-2008 I worked in one of the most aggressive commercial environments there is. My role as a recruitment consultant was 80% cold calling in am extremely saturated sales arena. Despite my own gentle soul, I found ways not only to compete, but to excel.

- Learn how to pinpoint the best customers for your practice
- Cost your treatments to ensure every treatment is profitable for both you and your customer
- Discover how to make every conversation into a potential sale lead without becoming a complete and utter pain in the a*s!
- Uncover the reasons why you are not closing sales so you never have to make the same mistakes again
- Create a growth environment where you plan success and always find yourself stepping into it

If you are working with essential oils, and you want to make a good living for it, then you need to learn to sell. What's more, if you are going to say "selling doesn't work on my customers"....then you have simply been taught to do it wrongly.

My dream is to see aromatherapy at the forefront of medicine. I need an army of gifted healers to achieve that. Consider yourself to be my newest recruit and I am going to drill you till you are the slickest, subtlest and most effective marketeer there is. You have the knowledge to make people better, now let me give you the business prowess to heal even more people than you have ever done before.

The Secret Healer has stress in her sights and she's about to make a killing. Listen carefully...she has much to tell you. £1.99 / $2.99

www.thesecrethealer.co.uk

www.buildyourownreality.com

Works Cited

(2014). Retrieved 11 21, 2014, from Leiseke.com: http://lieske.com/channels/5e-spleen.htm

Al-Chalabi, A., Delamont, R. S., & Tu, M. R. (2011). *The Brain (Beginners Guides)*. Oneworld Publications (academic). Kindle Edition. .

Berkers, E. (2013). *Chakras/Introduction* . Retrieved 11 21, 2014, from Eclectic Energies: http://www.eclecticenergies.com/chakras/introduction.php

Bruce, J. (2014). *The Aura*. Build Your Own Reality.

Bruce, J. (1994). *The Garden of Eden* . Magdelena Press.

Damasio, A. (2008). *Descartes Error: : Emotion, Reason and the Human Brain* . Random House. Kindle Edition.

Damasio, A. (2011). *Self Comes to Mind: Constructing the Conscious Brain* . Random House. Kindle Edition.

Field T1, H.-R. M. (2005). *Cortisol decreases and serotonin and dopamine increase following massage therapy*. Retrieved 11 21, 2014, from Pubmed: http://www.ncbi.nlm.nih.gov/pubmed/16162447

J, Y. (2014, 05 14). *Limonene inhibits methamphetamine-induced locomotor activity via regulation of 5-HT neuronal function and dopamine release*. Retrieved 11 21, 2014, from Pubmed: http://www.ncbi.nlm.nih.gov/pubmed/24462212

Jonathan E. Sherin, M. P. (2011, 09). *Post-traumatic stress disorder: the neurobiological impact of psychological trauma*. Retrieved 11 06, 2014, from Pubmed.com: http://www.ncbi.nlm.nih.gov/pmc/articles/PMC3182008/

Jones, E. A. (2012). *Awaken to Healing Fragrance: The Power of Essential Oil Therapy* . North Atlantic Books. Kindle Edition. .

Kang BN1, H. S. (2013). *Regulation of serotonin-induced trafficking and migration of eosinophils.* Retrieved 11 22, 2014, from Pubmed: http://www.ncbi.nlm.nih.gov/pubmed/23372779

Kent, N. (2009-2014). *Mind Body Connection Glossary.* Retrieved 11 22, 2014, from My Holistic Healing : http://www.my-holistic-healing.com/mind-body-connection-glossary.html

Lis-Balcan, M. (1997). *Essential oils and 'aromatherapy': their modern role in healing.* Retrieved 11 22, 2014, from Pubmed: http://www.ncbi.nlm.nih.gov/pubmed/9519666

Ltd, S. n. (2009). *Emotions and the Organs.* Retrieved 21 11, 2014, from Shen- Nong: http://www.shen-nong.com/eng/principles/sevenemotions.html

Lv XN1, L. Z. (2013, 07 14). *Aromatherapy and the central nerve system (CNS): therapeutic mechanism and its associated genes.* Retrieved 11 21, 2014, from Pub Med: http://www.ncbi.nlm.nih.gov/pubmed/23531112

Medicine, S. L. (2004-2014). *Emotions and the Organs.* Retrieved 11 21, 2014, from Sacred Lotus.com: http://www.sacredlotus.com/go/foundations-chinese-medicine/get/causes-illness-7-emotions

Miller, J. (n.d.). *I wasn't ready for the smell.* Retrieved 11 22, 2014, from PTSD Soldiers perspective:

http://ptsdasoldiersperspective.blogspot.co.uk/2013/10/i-wasnt-ready-for-smell.html#comment-form

Myss, C. (2010). *Anatomy of The Spirit*. Random House. Kindle Edition.

Noontil, A. (1996). *The Body is the Barometer of The Soul*. Annette Noontil.

Palkovits M, E. R. (1987, 02). *Distribution and possible origin of beta-endorphin and ACTH in discrete brainstem nuclei of rats*. Retrieved 11 06, 2014, from Pubmed.com: http://www.ncbi.nlm.nih.gov/pubmed/3033542

Perry N1, P. E. (2006). *Aromatherapy in the management of psychiatric disorders: clinical and neuropharmacological perspectives*. Retrieved 11 21, 2014, from Pubmed: http://www.ncbi.nlm.nih.gov/pubmed/16599645

Peters MA1, W. A. (2014, 09 22). *Dopamine and serotonin regulate tumor behavior by affecting angiogenesis*. Retrieved 11 22, 2014, from Pubmed.com: http://www.ncbi.nlm.nih.gov/pubmed/25269824

Phd, C. P. (2012). *Molecules Of Emotion: Why You Feel The Way You Feel* . Simon & Schuster UK. Kindle Edition.

The Organ-Emotion Link. (Not Known). Retrieved 11 21, 2014, from Sahej.com: http://www.sahej.com/organ-emotion_printready.html

The Primary, secondary and tertiary emotions. (1998-2014). Retrieved 11 22, 2014, from Alley Dog. com: http://www.alleydog.com/topics/emotion.php#ixzz3JAjZ8e8s

Worwood, V. A. (1993). *Aromantics*. Bantam Books.

Worwood, V. A. *The Fragrant Mind.* 1997: Bantam.

Disclaimer

by SEQ Legal

(1)   Introduction

This disclaimer governs the use of this book. [By using this book, you accept this disclaimer in full. / We will ask you to agree to this disclaimer before you can access the book.]

(2)   Credit

This disclaimer was created using an SEQ Legal template.

(3)   No advice

The book contains information about aromatherapy and the use of essential oils.The information is not advice, and should not be treated as such.

[You must not rely on the information in the book as an alternative to qualified medical advice from a health professional. advice from an appropriately qualified professional. If you have any specific questions about any medical matter you should consult an appropriately qualified professional.]

[If you think you may be suffering from any medical condition you should seek immediate medical attention. You should never delay seeking medical advice, disregard medical advice, or discontinue medical treatment because of information in the book.]

(4)   No representations or warranties

To the maximum extent permitted by applicable law and subject to section 6 below, we exclude all representations, warranties, undertakings and guarantees relating to the book.

Without prejudice to the generality of the foregoing paragraph, we do not represent, warrant, undertake or guarantee:

that the information in the book is correct, accurate,

complete or non-misleading;

that the use of the guidance in the book will lead to any particular outcome or result; or

in particular, that by using the guidance in the book you will heal disease or work in any way as a cure for illness.

(5)   Limitations and exclusions of liability

The limitations and exclusions of liability set out in this section and elsewhere in this disclaimer: are subject to section 6 below; and govern all liabilities arising under the disclaimer or in relation to the book, including liabilities arising in contract, in tort (including negligence) and for breach of statutory duty.

We will not be liable to you in respect of any losses arising out of any event or events beyond our reasonable control.

We will not be liable to you in respect of any business losses, including without limitation loss of or damage to profits, income, revenue, use, production, anticipated savings, business, contracts, commercial opportunities or goodwill.

We will not be liable to you in respect of any loss or corruption of any data, database or software.

We will not be liable to you in respect of any special, indirect or consequential loss or damage.

(6) Exceptions

Nothing in this disclaimer shall: limit or exclude our liability for death or personal injury resulting from negligence; limit or exclude our liability for fraud or fraudulent misrepresentation; limit any of our liabilities in any way that is not permitted under applicable law; or exclude any of our liabilities that may not be excluded under applicable law.

(7) Severability

If a section of this disclaimer is determined by any court or other competent authority to be unlawful and/or unenforceable, the other sections of this disclaimer continue in effect.

If any unlawful and/or unenforceable section would be lawful or enforceable if part of it were deleted, that part will be deemed to be deleted, and the rest of the section will continue in effect.

(8)   Law and jurisdiction

This disclaimer will be governed by and construed in accordance with English law, and any disputes relating to this disclaimer will be subject to the exclusive jurisdiction of the courts of England and Wales.

(9)   Our details

In this disclaimer, "we" means (and "us" and "our" refer to) [*Elizabeth Ashley*] of [*SY8 1LQ*].

CPSIA information can be obtained at www.ICGtesting.com
Printed in the USA
LVOW11s1707300715

448252LV00021B/852/P